MEDICAL PARADOXES

MEDICAL PARADOXES

Contradictions in current medicine

DR FRANCISCO KERDEL-VEGAS

Translated from the Spanish by
Kate Auckland

PUBLICACIONES VIOLETA, 2016
como homenaje al autor · as a tribute to the author

First published in the Spanish language as *Paradojas Médicas* by
Cognitio in 2014
www.cognitiobooks.com

First published in Great Britain in 2016 by
Publicaciones Violeta, London

A CIP catalogue record for this book is available
from the British Library.

ISBN: 978-0-9955415-0-4

Designed and typeset in Haarlemmer by Libanus Press, Marlborough
Printed and bound in Great Britain by Hampton Printing (Bristol) Ltd

To medical students all over the world who will be challenged by many and new paradoxes, and on whose moral integrity the future of our noble profession largely depends.

THE AUTHOR

The English edition of this book is due to the combined efforts of friends who are convinced of its value to medics, students of medicine and the general public. I would like to thank José Alvarez Stelling for his leadership and financial support, without which this publication would not have been possible; Carlota Páez de Wigglesworth for her encouragement and loyalty; Alfred W. Kopf for his academic input and comments; Charles Pasternak for his foreword; and Kate Auckland for her translation and project management. I am eternally grateful to them.

DR FRANCISCO KERDEL-VEGAS

CONTENTS

FOREWORD

PROFESSOR CHARLES PASTERNAK

President of the Oxford International Biomedical Centre

I was fortunate to meet Francisco Kerdel-Vegas during the early 1990s when he was serving as Venezuelan Ambassador in London. I had just founded the Oxford International Biomedical Centre (OIBC) and was looking for potential Patrons of this organisation. Kerdel-Vegas – the most eclectic of physicians – fitted the role perfectly: luckily for me and the institution, he accepted. We continued our close friendship throughout the following years during which he moved to Paris as Venezuelan Ambassador to France and to UNESCO. I was much impressed with my colleague's diplomatic skills: medically-trained envoys are thin on the ground

Francisco Kerdel-Vegas is equally qualified to write this compendium of 100 medical paradoxes. *Paradojas Médicas. Contradicciones de la medicina actual* encompasses and up-dates a series of articles written by him on the topic during 2004 and 2005. Kerdel-Vegas begins his *magnum opus* with an account of the first patient who came to see him after he set up a private medical practice in Caracas at the age of 26. The patient had no obvious symptoms, but Kerdel-Vegas's intuition suggested to him that the young man sitting in front of him might be suffering from early-stage leprosy. Back in 1954 this was as taboo a subject as homosexuality or insanity. Kerdel-Vegas cautiously explained the necessary procedures to verify such a diagnosis. Not only was the young doctor's hunch confirmed, but he was then able to successfully eradicate the dreaded infection. The patient is now a healthy grandfather in his late eighties.*

Such perspicacity remained with Kerdel-Vegas for the next sixty years, and is evident now in this fascinating work. Before describing each paradox in turn, the author presents a short synopsis of the history of medicine from Hippocrates to the use of Viagra for male impotence in 1998. Among the more important discoveries he rightly highlights the isolation of penicillin in 1941. The story is familiar to most readers. What is less well-known is that the Oxford researchers were not the only ones working on penicillin at that time. A group of scientists at the Netherlands Yeast and Spirit Factory in Delft had, by 1943, also realised the implications of Fleming's 1928 discovery that a mould called *Penicillium* extrudes material that apparently inhibits the growth of certain bacteria. In secrecy, under the noses of the German occupiers, they began to purify extracts of such moulds (the fact that one of their associates was a Jewish physician in fear of transportation to the Theresienstadt extermination camp did not help). In order to disguise their aim, the scientists gave their isolates an innocuous name: Bacinol. By June 1944, as the allied armies were landing in Normandy, the Dutch researchers were successfully treating infected rabbits and mice with Bacinol. In April 1945, when the group were finally able to lay their hands on US-manufactured tablets of penicillin, they showed that Bacinol is indeed penicillin.[1] Perhaps in a second edition of *Paradojas Médicas*, the author might include a 101st Paradox: "Published vs. unpublished investigation" or "Medical research in a free vs. an oppressed society".

All hundred of the Paradoxes make interesting reading, and in this short Foreword I can do justice to no more than a handful. I liked the

---

* The author relates this story in full in his Introduction.

12th Paradox: "Doctors vs. Lawyers" because it reminded me of Jess M. Brallier's 1992 book *Lawyers and Other Reptiles*. The 55th Paradox: "The contribution of doctors to medicine vs. Doctors' contributions to other branches of the cultural universe" is particularly pertinent: is being an ambassador not a contribution to the cultural universe? Some Paradoxes, such as the 63rd Paradox: "Science fiction vs. Medical fiction", are light-hearted. Others, like the 66th Paradox: "Prolongation of life vs. Quality of life" or the 88th Paradox: "Cancer treatment: Surgery vs. Radiotherapy vs. Chemotherapy" go to the very essence of today's medical predicaments. I particularly appreciate the 76th Paradox: 'Diseases of deficiency vs. Diseases of affluence' since it sits easily alongside a publication based on a symposium organised by the Oxford International Biomedical Centre[2] of which, as mentioned, the author is a Patron.

Medical Paradoxes is an enjoyable read for two reasons. First, because the author is an accomplished writer with a light touch. Second, because his erudition is as extensive as his medical knowledge. Readers of this book may find some of the author's paradoxes surprising, others less so. Perhaps I may take the liberty of pointing out that science itself – as rigorous and logical a discipline as any – also throws up the occasional paradox. The developmental biologist Lewis Wolpert, whom Kerdel-Vegas quotes in another context, calls it *The Unnatural Nature of Science*.[3]

REFERENCES

1   Marlene Burns and Piet WM van Dijck, "The development of the penicillin production process in Delft, the Netherlands, during the Second World War under Nazi occupation". *Adv. Appl. Microbiol*, 51: 185-200 (2002)

2   *Access Not Excess. The search for better nutrition* (ed. Charles Pasternak; Smith-Gordon, St Ives, Cambs, 2011)

3   Lewis Wolpert, *The Unnatural Nature of Science* (Faber, London, 1992)

INTRODUCTION

I had just returned from three years in the United States specialising in dermatology. Following in the footsteps of other doctors in my family (two uncles and my maternal grandfather), I was attempting to carve a path for myself and earn my living as a doctor. I had established my private surgery in a tiny rented apartment in the city centre (next to a large private clinic and a big brewery) and was endeavouring to attract my first patients in order to maintain that difficult balance between practice in the public sector (in hospitals and faculties of medicine), which at the time generated only a token salary, and private sector practice, from which the professional earned their real living; dividing my time wisely, with mornings spent on the first and afternoons dedicated to the second.

Never does time pass more slowly than for a doctor who has recently begun his private medical practice and is waiting nervously for the doorbell to ring in announcement of his first patient. Time spent wondering whether you will be able to pay the rent, electricity and telephone bills, and nurse and receptionist salaries, the bare minimum required to launch oneself into the adventure of opening your own surgery. My uncle, Doctor Martín Vegas, had generously agreed to my request to put his name on the apartment door plaque and come out of retirement to accompany me for a few hours a week and thereby attract potential patients. This undoubtedly would have occurred given his fame and prestige if people had only been aware that he was there and available, but he didn't wish to advertise (classified adverts in the press required the local Medical College's approval), perhaps in consideration of his old associates at the prominent clinic in the capital from which he had retired some time before.

What causes a patient to consult a novice such as I was back in 1954? I still ask myself that.

The fact is that amongst the first ten patients who dared to try their luck with this newcomer is T. F. (name of course invented to protect his confidentiality). Tomy is a young man of around 26 years old (the same age that I was at the time), handsome, entrepreneurial, kind, talkative, married with three children very close in age, living with his in-laws and working for a business belonging to the brother of his mother-in-law. We are not just similar in age, civil state and paternity, but also in that we depend on the generosity of our in-laws to look after our families. Tomy has stiffness in his little fingers and ring fingers and has been treated by a distinguished doctor in the capital (one of my respected teachers) without any apparent improvement. He comes to the surgery accompanied by his mother-in-law and recommended by family contacts who think that a doctor recently arrived from the North will perhaps be able to offer new curative medicine.

Almost as soon as I see him I have a suspected diagnosis, what a teacher of mine would have called a "diagnóstico de las cocineras" (or cook's diagnosis), in other words glaringly obvious to a trained mind.

His mother-in-law, an executive, forceful and domineering, married to a man much older than her, speaks for him and explains that they want to try something new as the treatment prescribed had not had any results.

As my tentative diagnosis, which I keep *in pectore*, is nothing more, nothing less than the most terrible of its kind – leprosy – I mentally prepare a suitable strategy to manage such a difficult situation.

The clinical examination confirms my suspicions, palpation reveals an ulnar nerve that is considerably increased in size, such as I had been taught presents itself in tuberculoid leprosy. The consequences of a neural invasion of Hansen's bacillus are already showing in his hand.

The first thing I have to do is carefully question the patient alone, without his mother-in-law. As I need to carry out several additional examinations (sensitivity, biopsy, etc.), I offer him another appointment.

Unfortunately his mother-in-law accompanies him once again. I have no other choice than to re-examine him and assign him another appointment. Third time lucky and Tomy turns up at my surgery alone.

The strategy to follow is very direct. The first step is to make him understand little by little that we think he has leprosy. For example, it is known and commented upon by the general public that there is an endemic focus of leprosy in Colonia Tovar (a touristy village in the mountains near to Caracas, inhabited by descendants of German colonists). For this reason I ask him most emphatically if he frequently visits there. As I notice that he doesn't pay any attention to this turn of questioning, I ask him more directly if he has had any contact with a leper. On denying this, I anxiously ask him again, saying that I suspect that he may have leprosy whilst trying to calm him by saying that it's just a possibility that I have to discount. My uncle Martín Vegas told me of the tragic case of a patient who committed suicide after having been diagnosed with leprosy. He taught me how human beings can slowly get used to the harshest of realities if the truth is administered in small, calculated and progressive doses. Just like in the well-known tale of the frog that dies in a pot of boiling oil, as the temperature increases gradually, little by little he is able to tolerate every increase in temperature until the final outcome.

After various visits and supplementary examinations and the indispensible psychological preparation of days in suspense, I consider the ground to be suitably prepared to reveal the harsh truth:

3

"Tomy, the disease affecting you is leprosy. But leprosy these days, in 1954, is a curable disease that doesn't even require isolation," I am quick to inform him. "However, as tales and prejudices about the incurability and contagious nature of this terrible affliction persist, it is imperative that this situation remain exclusively, without any exception, between you and me. My passion to keep this information secret is such that even in your clinical history in my own surgery your diagnosis will be hidden under a codename that only I know, to avoid the indiscreet eyes of those not bound by the Hippocratic Oath finding out the truth (like the nurse or receptionist)", I add immediately. He listens to me with hollow eyes, in a state of profound and dumb sadness. "I repeat: the illness when adequately treated is curable and in contrast to a short time ago does not require isolation. Moreover, fortunately, the variety of leprosy that you have is the most benign and should not affect your daily routine, your work or your family relationships" I insist, trying to give the greatest authority and conviction to what I am saying. He watches me in incredulous silence and takes time to answer. When he does, after seconds that seem like minutes, with a shaking voice and great apathy he says the following (more or less): "Supposing that what you say doctor is true, there is a difficulty that is impossible to overcome; keeping the nature of my illness a secret between you and me. The relationship that I have sworn to maintain with my wife obliges me to tell her the truth." I answer that this seems a noble and admirable position, but that in this specific case it is not advisable. I observe that it greatly bothers him that I doubt the loyalty of his wife, and so it is that I explain to him that apart from other motives, it is a sure way of protecting her from infinite unnecessary doubts and suffering. I see that I have lost this battle and as I don't want to lose the war, I retreat and hastily offer a conciliatory proposition. I ask him to think about the matter for a week, without saying anything to his wife, and come back

4

after this period to tell me his decision. After considering this for what seems a long time, he agrees to my proposal.

Tomy was undoubtedly less aware of the stigmas of leprosy than I was even before I became a dermatologist or even a doctor or student of medicine. As a child, I discerned from vague and broken whispers the tale of a relative with leprosy, and the sufferings of their whole family to shut them away in a room in the house, avoiding contact with their loved ones, and above all preventing anybody from revealing the situation, which would have had unpredictable social consequences, for urban society at that time was rather narrow-minded and judgemental. Perhaps, and this I could never discuss with my uncle as it was a taboo subject in the family, this tale led to him becoming interested in leprosy and attempting to improve the terrible living conditions of those afflicted. My mother used to tell us how, as an unmarried woman, she would translate scientific articles on leprosy from French to Spanish for her brother (my uncle Martín), and was left tormented by descriptions of its development and consequences, how the skin of limbs was often poked with a pin to determine if there was an absence of feeling to thereby detect the illness. But in reality, it wasn't until almost at the end of my medical studies when as part of an internship for the Chair of Dermatology we visited the leper colony of Cabo Blanco in Maiquetía (knocked down many years ago to make way for the expansion of the Simón Bolívar International Airport). There I had the opportunity to examine dozens of lepers and observe the horrible mutilations and deformities of the dreaded disease. At that time, in 1950, I came to understand the true significance of the magnitude and intensity of such a destructive and incapacitating chronic illness as leprosy, the terrible reality of the isolation and ostracism to which those human beings were condemned for life, without any hope of a curative treatment, which at that that time was nonexistent. The vocation and sacrifice of the doctors, nurses and auxiliary staff who were so dedicated to tending to their patients awoke in me an admiration and respect that has only increased with the passing of the years.

Ever since I can remember I have been undoubtedly aware of the significance of being diagnosed with leprosy, having heard and at times read so many tales about it. There was the Leper King of Jerusalem who used a silver mask to hide his gradual destruction from the disease during the Crusades. Or the moving story of Father Damien of Molokai who was dedicated to the care of lepers in Hawaii and who eventually contracted and died from the disease himself; he was canonised as a Saint in 2009.

I reflected on all of this, that I couldn't ask Tomy to objectively measure the risks to his future and his position in his recently formed family if anybody, with the exception of the doctor and his patient, were to find out that he had leprosy. At the time, effective sulphone treatment for leprosy was recent and relatively unknown. Even when cases of bacterial resistance to this treatment later appeared, they would be overcome in turn by the multidrug therapy that is still valid to this day.

Today I ask myself if Tomy in his naïve and partial ignorance of all of the terrible prejudices that existed (many of which persist) would come to realise what could happen to him, his marriage, his family, his job, his future. Would he consider the possibility that his young and attractive wife would have nightmares sleeping next to a leper, or even that in consideration of the highly contagious nature of the disease would try to keep him away from his children? How would his in-laws, with whom he was living, react when he was barely at the start of being economically productive? What would his employer and his co-workers think if they found out about the situation?

It's likely that he didn't ask himself any of this, at least not with the intensity (and authority?) that I did, but my conscience obliged me to think of the different possibilities and protect my naïve and young patient by considering the worst of them as real. Undoubtedly the advisable thing to do was to keep the secret of his disease exclusively between us.

In perfect knowledge of the fact that in medicine there exists no absolute truth, but conscious as I was of the doubts that tormented my patient, I said to him:

"If you swear to me that you will never reveal the secret of your disease to another person and that you are going to strictly follow the treatment and rules that I will set for you, I will take on the responsibility of treating you until you are cured, without you being submitted to isolation, separated from your family or any other alteration in your daily life, and without your wife or children running the risk of being infected by the disease."

He dutifully answered me that although he didn't completely share my opinion, he accepted my better judgement based on my scientific knowledge of the matter and agreed to the deal.

Within a short time I arranged a small surgical intervention to free his ulnar nerve and improve the functioning of his hand, which was carried out by a skilful surgeon with extensive experience in leper colonies, and which had the anticipated success.

Having strictly followed his treatment he was cured from his illness and in turn released as my patient.

Now that more than half a century has passed since that episode in my life, I have on occasion seen Tomy, his wife, children and grandchildren socially and it is clear that he is an honourable citizen, head of the family, father and grandfather to a large family, successful executive of a small business, clearly happy and fulfilled. This leads me to think, in fact it obliges me to meditate, on what would have happened if I had acted differently to how I did, with the determination and strictness to

7

which on rare occasions I have had to resort during my professional practice.

I am convinced that Tomy never realised the gravity of his situation, the severity of his illness or the perilous consequences of all of the prejudices that Hansen's disease has accumulated throughout history. In other words, Tomy never completely realised the significance of my strong position and behaviour as a doctor, something to which I never aspired, conscious of how in correct professional practice one shouldn't seek the applause and gratitude of the patient and their relatives, but place their interests alone above all other considerations. It is good and holy if both coincide, as sometimes occurs, but if that isn't the case we must accept that the most important thing is to be at peace with our own conscience. Only God knows the happiness and fulfilment that I feel when I see Tomy happy and fulfilled: I as a doctor, him as a citizen and father to his family.

NOTE: In his considerable experience, the distinguished Argentine-Canadian philosopher and writer Mario Bunge suggested that I begin the English edition of *Medical Paradoxes* by narrating an interesting clinical case, for which reason I chose to expand upon the story briefly described in Paradox 34, which demonstrates the reach of influence of a doctor in the life and future of his or her patients. It is clear that most of the time the drama narrated here does not manifest itself with such intensity, but to a greater or lesser degree a doctor's good judgement can determine the future of their patients, something that they must always keep in mind.

PROLOGUE

RAFAEL MUCI-MENDOZA

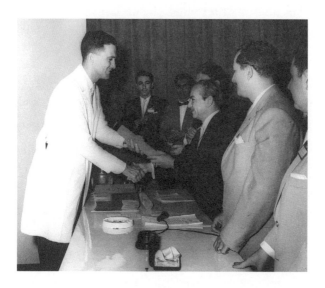

This photo shows the seventieth anniversary of the Hospital Vargas in Caracas (July 1961) in which this book's author receives one of the prizes given on that occasion from Mr Alejandro Oropeza Castillo, Governor of the Federal District (hidden in this photo).
Photograph donated to Dr Rafael Muci-Mendoza by the children of Dr Blas Bruni-Celli.

In the turbulent environment of medicine in both the last and present centuries thus far, I take it as a duty of great honour and a delicious obligation to serve as herald for *Medical Paradoxes* written by academic and friend, Doctor Francisco Kerdel-Vegas; a task that I accept with considerable gratitude.

Ever since my first contact some years ago with the 100 Paradoxes that form this book, they have, in many respects, represented for me a "departure point", both stimulating and entertaining, for diverse aspects of medicine on which I had neither the time nor place to reflect. The leap from one subject to another indicates the tightly woven nature of these issues, revealing strange anomalies in the intimate fibre of medicine. The Paradoxes do not suffer when the author offers a flash of humour and mischief, making them all the more palatable to the reader who is always given much on which to meditate, learn and admire.

For the good of his colleagues, patients and the general public, Kerdel-Vegas has published the juicy fruits of his studies and experience in a rarely visited area of medicine; paradoxes, concepts that are at times irreconcilable and at other times compatible. In fact, each paradox vies to be a subject worthy of careful reflection in its own right. One of the main points of which the author convinces us is that all the topics raised in this book are, in fact, a single issue. They represent multiple and different paths that lead to a common centre, which, in my opinion, corresponds to the modern philosophical culture of medicine. Understanding the fundamental problems of medicine has always been in general human interest and therefore, must be understood by us, medicine's devotees, and by the greater public.

In this book, you will encounter Kerdel-Vegas, with the rebelliousness that marks his still youthful impetus, seizing the lance and battling through the paradoxes that are present but forgotten in our daily journey as doctors; these paradoxes surround our field of medicine where the injustices and errors borne of our scientific past and present are not only perceived more keenly than anywhere else, but also those other wonders that must be counted, analysed and admired. His book facilitates an understanding and acceptance of the limitations of medicine as a study of life, offering a better comprehension of reality by discerning between what can be controlled and what cannot, enabling the acceptance of human misery, whilst at the same time appreciating the beauty of life and the practice of medicine.

These 100 Paradoxes, where, I consider, almost everything – light shared with darkness, the obvious with the hidden, the equal with the different– is of such great practical importance that I do not doubt that the book should form part of the medical curriculum, especially when students begin to make contact and amateur efforts with their first patients and the illnesses that afflict them. The Paradoxes are an embodiment of moderation and implicit good advice. They are an antidote to the omnipotence that so often enthrals modern medicine, which is dazzled by technology, and will help to redress the balance, although not always.

Now we must focus our attention briefly on the author of this book. Kerdel-Vegas is first and foremost a doctor, but he is much more than that, not simply a medical practitioner, he possesses that particular quality that encapsulates everything a doctor should be. Far back in the past, and more recently in the present, I have been witness to his career and I can testify to his love for work and analytical reading, his astuteness and the intense preparation as a universal doctor that has led to his preferential and respected position within national medicine. He is a doctor of both literary and scientific culture, a wise man of life experience, a man of letters, a humanist, a dermatologist and author of numerous scientific works related to the skin, and a book co-authored with an eminent figure in dermatology at a worldwide level, Doctor George Clinton Andrews, entitled *Diseases of the Skin,* (I own the two volumes of its fourth edition in Spanish); a product of his frenzied scientific activity. Furthermore, he is one of those people concerned by the growing problem of the Venezuelan talent drain and has been dedicated for some time to preventing the incremental increase in the number of highly qualified individuals who, for many reasons, are leaving the country. He has sought, confronted and reconciled them once again with their homeland. The UNESCO TALVEN programme, *Talento Venezolano en el Exterior* (Venezuelan Talent Abroad), has grown from his concern for such an important issue.

He was a first-rate and excellent Ambassador for Venezuela, representing us with great integrity in the United Kingdom, in France and then UNESCO, a zealous observer of his duty to promote both the Venezuelan people and our national science. Furthermore, his restless and inquiring mind, rich with ideas, has led him, decisively and with great expertise, to venture successfully into virtual journalism. Assisted by a highly learned team, he established the Spanish language health website/blog *Bitácora Médica*. It is an essential source of information and doctors who visits its pages once will return again and again to quench their thirst for knowledge and their need to be up to date, whilst at the same time enjoying themselves. Even more recently, his fascination with modern technology, of which he is well-informed, convinced us of the benefits of technological gadgets, Amazon's "Kindle" or the electronic book; a sort of portable, travelling library, lightweight and wonderful for amassing science, literature, art, poetry, music, videos and Wi-Fi, with the capacity for 1,400 titles and weighing just 345 grams. And yet, whilst all of this may be true . . . I do still miss the smell of a new book.

And here I must finish, so as not to delay your reading of Doctor Kerdel-Vegas' book any further; a simple book of complete scientific architecture that fills a gap in our medical literature and which I devoured with the joy of a dedicated fan.

PREFACE

In 2004 and 2005, I published a series of articles under the title "*Grandes Paradojas de la Medicina Actual*" ("The Great Paradoxes of Current Medicine") which drew medical colleagues' and students' attention to what are collectively called "paradoxes" (defined by Collins Dictionary as "a person or thing exhibiting apparently contradictory characteristics"). I grouped together diverse subjects with evident discrepancies, inconsistencies and contradictions, which, thanks to the interest of its president at the time, Dr José Enrique López, were later assembled in an extensive chapter of Volume II of the *Colección Razetti de la Academia Nacional de Medicina de Venezuela* (The Razetti Collection of the National Academy of Medicine of Venezuela). They also incorporated two very interesting commentaries by academics Augusto León and J. M. Avilán-Rovira. As I am convinced of the importance of spreading this type of information amongst the general public, this new edition is an attempt to divulge it more widely, so that the dilemmas that run through doctors' minds every time they attend to their patients are understood more thoroughly. The content has been corrected and updated and, taking advantage of current technological advances, is now presented simultaneously in printed and digital versions.

Although a great part of this book maintains its original format, I have tried to incorporate new statistical figures, especially demographic figures, thereby permitting the reader to evaluate the changes of the last few years.

When I asked various friends to read the manuscript, their names are mentioned on page 281, some of them not only suggested spelling and syntax changes but also made the additional effort of commenting on the content by including their own remarks. As awakening the curiosity and creativity of readers in relation to these medical Paradoxes has always been the aim of this book, with their consent and my gratitude for their efforts I am including their comments as an Addendum.

In order to facilitate the reader's understanding of the relation in time of the different people mentioned, in this edition I have incorporated in brackets their dates of birth and death (this last one only if relevant). Brief notes on persons referred to in the main body of the text are given at the foot of the page, indicated by an asterisk.

PRELIMINARY CONSIDERATIONS

"Give a soul to medicine, a conscience to science."
JEAN BERNARD (1907–2006)

I don't believe there is a better way to sum up the principal concerns of medicine and science in our time than with these two ideas, chosen as the epigraph for this book. They were written by the French doctor, academic and writer Jean Bernard (1907–2006), whose opinion essentially focuses on the sphere of morality and ethics.

Medicine's origins are lost in the mists of time, the antiquity of our reliance on medicine is confirmed by the frequency with which we refer our problems to a doctor, priest or lawyer, for they facilitate our understanding of the control of the natural, supernatural and relationships on society.

There is a school of thought that establishes a direct relationship between monotheistic religions and medicine, for according to Western tradition the idea of a single God has a deterministic effect on biomedicine (a fashionable term used to describe contemporary scientific medicine). To a certain extent this legitimises the idea of one sole universal underlying truth, or in other words, a universal paradigm (Paul Unschuld*).

General discontent with the lack of new "medical miracles" to cure degenerative diseases in old age has meant that in recent years we have seen the emergence of new medical fashions that have swelled the ranks of the well-established unorthodox movements of homeopathy,

* Paul Unschuld, German medical historian (1943–)

osteopathy, podiatry, and chiropractic, practices such as "holism", herbalism, acupuncture, aromatherapy, and numerous other titles that fall under the "alternative medicine" description.

Medicine, in so much that it is a discipline that works simultaneously with science and art, is deeply connected to the morality and ethics of its age. Morals are more flexible and vary with the times; ethics feed off permanent values and basic principles.

There is no doubt in my mind of the many and important benefits that medicine provides to our daily lives; something which acquired more importance in my generation, that is to say the second half of the twentieth century, in which new medicines and surgical procedures permitting the cure or control of certain illnesses were discovered, leading to statistics that irrefutably prove the achievements of medicine of our day. Not only are people living longer, but they are enjoying better health, this is so clear, well-known and accepted by public opinion that taxpayers pressurise and oblige politicians to multiply their expenditure on the health industry, which has come to be the largest in the world.

To gain a valid assessment of the Venezuelan health sector, we have only to consult the health expenditure page on the World Health Organisation's website (for 2001), where raw figures show that Venezuela matches Haiti as the Latin American country that spends the least on health in the region (a dead heat between Venezuela and Haiti with 4.2% of the public and private GDP (gross domestic product)). This is something that any sensible government should immediately correct.

The country with the highest health expenditure is the United States with 13% of its GDP spent on health, followed by Nicaragua (12.2%), Germany (10.6%), Switzerland (10.4%), Argentina (10.3%), Lebanon (9.8%), France (9.6%), Israel (9.5%), Colombia (9.3%), Canada (9.2 %) and Cuba (9.1%). This group invests more than 9% of their GDP on health; as we can observe from these eleven countries, six are developed nations and five are undeveloped, of the second group four are Latin American and one could say that, at least in this sector, they have made a laudable and perhaps recent effort to improve the health of their population and thereby attempt to leave the poor hygiene / illness / poverty / hunger vicious circle.

I asked my dear friend and colleague José Felix Oletta (Professor of Internal Medicine and ex-Minister of Health and Social Welfare in Venezuela) to update these figures for the second edition of this book. I copy the information that he sent me below:

"The health expenditure trend in Venezuela is regressive, from 6% of the GDP in 2007 to 5.2% in 2011. Likewise, the expenditure on health in the public sector (as a percentage of total health expenditure) fell from 44.5% in 2007 to 36.7% in 2011. Source: the World Health Organisation's Global Health Expenditure Database (see http:// apps.who.int/nha/database).

Therefore, the private health expenditure of those people who pay for healthcare from their own pockets or via private insurance is greater than the Government's contributions; this indicates that health expenditure in Venezuela is increasingly unjust and affects population groups of the lowest socioeconomic conditions the most.

What does health expenditure consist of? According to the 2009 Encuesta Nacional de Presupuesto Familiar (National Survey on Family Budgets) the structure of household health consumption is fundamentally shaped by the following items: Medicines 47.3%; Therapeutic Apparatus and Equipment 5%; Medical and paramedical services 27.4% and Hospital Services 20.2%. The weighting of the aforementioned items varies according to the distribution of income levels in the population. If indeed medicines do constitute the item that is the greatest burden on household health expenditure, for the poorest 25% of the population (1st quartile) it represents 66.5% of health expenditure, for the second quartile it is 60.7% and for the third and fourth percentiles 57.7% and 41% respectively. Source: BCV (Banco Central de Venzuela). Preliminary figures IV National Survey on Family Budgets (2009); Salvato S. Añez E. (El financiamiento de la Salud. Integrar más que dividir (Funding Health. Integrate more than divide.), Encuentro de Organizaciones Sociales (Meeting of Social Organisations), UCAB (Universidad Católica Andrés Bello), UCV (Universidad Central de Venezuela) 2012."

As the distinguished and prolific British medical historian Roy Porter (1946–2002) maintained: "Never have people in the West lived so long, or been so healthy, and never have medical achievements been so great. Yet, paradoxically, rarely has medicine drawn such intense doubts and disapproval as today. No-one could deny that the medical breakthroughs of the past 50 years – the culmination of a long tradition of scientific medicine – have saved more lives than those of any era since the dawn of medicine." (Porter, 2006: 6)

This transformation and the substantial injection of funds that have occurred in very few years have not been without negative effect on the practice of our profession, which until a few years ago, as far as the economic landscape was concerned, carried on as a "homemade" or primitive industry, just as we were taught by our teachers, just as practised for decades. This has caused me to re-think the reason for the challenges faced on a daily basis in the unique doctor/patient relationship.

I write these words because, as Roy Porter suggests, we are children of Gutenberg (1395–1486), and we are trapped in a web of words, and because, as the Bible says, "In the beginning was the Word". When all is said and done we are the product of the religions of the book and its philosophy of the power of the written word.

I must admit from the outset that a summary such as I wish to present for the scrutiny of the medical class and the general public is damaged by my "historicism", if my belief that the study of history helps us to understand the present and even predict the future can be described as such. Living without this fundamental intellectual basis for our conduct would be like traversing deep into the ocean without a compass or marine chart.

Clearly we want to share these ideas with colleagues and, with their active participation, open up a debate that permits an objective evaluation of the current situation.

Attempting to ignore, sidestep, shun, avoid or postpone making decisions in the face of the challenging realities imposed by the impressive technological and economic development in the sphere of health sciences, with all the unavoidable pressures and direct interventions in professional medical practice, would undeniably be akin to the ostrich strategy of burying its head in the sand when faced with a crisis of magnitude.

The ideas expressed here have been studied, discussed and disseminated by numerous authors, doctors and lay people alike, for which reason I must state that I unequivocally share the evaluation of the distinguished North American medical writer Sherwin B. Nuland (1930–2014) when he stated: "No author writes alone. Whatever his degree of solitude, the silent influence of seemingly long-forgotten words are always at his elbow, and so are the men and women who spoke them; the reading and the talk of a lifetime converge on his pages. Filtered through the individuality of a writer's mind, the distant echoes of experience become ever more insistent until they make themselves known, and find form at his fingertips though they may never rise into full, unveiled consciousness." (Nuland, 1998: xi)

The daily practice of contemporary medicine presents numerous contradictions and paradoxes that are hard to interpret and even more complex to resolve, and which are worth identifying in order to draw the attention and interest of professionals. This is in no way an exhaustive list, nor is any particular hierarchy of importance anticipated, therefore the paradoxes are not numbered in order of importance or foreseeable consequence. I believe that it is important for the medical profession to periodically review these paradoxes, which will clearly change from time to time, with the continual, and at times explosive, evolution of the health sciences. This depends in large part on being able to maintain a high moral solvency in the practice of medicine, given its well-earned and age-old reputation based on gravitas, accolade, honour and integrity. A direct result of this is the high level of confidence and credibility enjoyed by the doctor, indispensable in any society in order to be able to practise their profession ideally. This privileged position that society has given us must not be violated or diminished, as it is the foundation of a transparent and fair relationship; on the one hand individually, between the patient and the treating doctor, and on the other collectively, between the medical profession and society.

These two concepts of confidence and credibility are fundamental in medical practice, which is why we must repeatedly insist on their importance and support ourselves with the opinion of reputable authors to reinforce it in our readers' minds.

As will be observed, these paradoxes, chosen at random and in no way a complete inventory, have a variety of characters; philosophical, ethical, moral, ontological, deontological, semiological, semantic, economic, administrative, procedural, cultural amongst others. However, what they have in common is an interest of a practical nature for the doctor in the practice of his or her profession.

Many of these paradoxes are intimately related to each other, given the nature of the problem being addressed and will eventually be able to be grouped.

The history of medicine

Medicine is as old as man's first appearance on our planet. It is thought that *Homo sapiens,* as such, evolved from superior primates some 100,000 – 120,000 years ago. However, we only have written proof (history) for 2500 years, which is what truly counts in documented evolution. In order to try to determine the influence of medicine on the development of our species during that considerable period of time for which we possess reliable information, it is therefore pertinent that we ask ourselves questions like the one that follows.

The contributions made by doctors

Which are the most significant contributions made by doctors to the benefit of humanity?

To answer this question we need to refer to the rather subjective evaluation attempted in 1978 by the American astrophysicist and writer Michael H. Hart (1932–). This was his evaluation of the influence of the significant – not always positive – actions, works, discoveries and innovations throughout history, those that affect the greatest number of people for the longest period of time, and the men responsible for them. They are listed from 1 to 100 in hierarchical order according to each one's relative importance and include the following doctors: Sigmund Freud (1856–1939; number 32 in the first edition of the book and later demoted to number 69 in the second edition in 1993), Alexander Fleming (1881–1955; number 45), John Locke (1632–1704; number 48), William Harvey (1578–1657; number 57), Joseph Lister (1827–1912; number 60), and Edward Jenner (1749–1823: number 72). In other words, only 6% of the total are doctors, in fact to be more precise, perhaps even only 5% if we exclude Locke, for although he practised medicine throughout his life, he achieved the immortality of this list through his contributions to philosophy and not medicine. To be fair, the contributions to medical science made by non-doctors were perhaps even more important than those of the doctors, of these we cannot fail to mention the achievements of Louis Pasteur (1822–95; number 12), Charles Darwin (1809–82; number 17), Wilhelm Conrad Röntgen (1845–1923; number 73), and Gregory Pincus (1903–67; number 81).

Whichever way this list is analysed, it is clear that the contributions of these great men have given substantial form and content to the world in which we live. Of the six doctors, five were British and one Austrian. Of the non-doctor scientists one was French, one British, one German and the other American.

The decision of who to include in the list followed by an even harder classification is a greatly interesting and significant intellectual exercise, but one that is also inevitably highly subjective. As the popular proverb says, *"no son todos los que están, ni están todos los que son"* which roughly translates as "not everybody who should be is on here, and some people who are on it shouldn't be"; undoubtedly one of the greatest absentees is Hippocrates.

This was acknowledged by the author in the second edition of his book, published in 1993, this time by a prestigious publishing house with the capacity for universal circulation and marketing (Simon & Schuster of New York). In a simple list of 200 people, of which only the first 100 are accompanied by a mini-biography, he includes another three doctors in alphabetical order: Galen (130–210), Hippocrates (460 BC–370 BC) and Ivan Pavlov (1849–1936).

There are a number of great benefactors for the human enjoyment of health and wellbeing who remain unknown, some of them completely anonymous or very poorly remembered. Let us take an example. Who remembers the inventor of eyeglasses or spectacles? We know from *The Wealth and Poverty of Nations* by Professor David Landes that this invention took place in the Italian city of Pisa around the year

1306. The inventor of this great discovery (possibly a simple artisan, whose exact name we do not know) attached polished glass to a metal framework that was supported by the nose and ears (the corrective properties in vision were already known, for it is said that Nero used a monocle carved out of emerald to read). With this simple invention this benefactor to humanity doubled the visual working life of millions of workers, and allowed those who read to continue reading for the rest of their lives.

The paternity of discoveries

It is also appropriate to remember here that very often just one person capitalises upon the credit for a discovery, when in truth, and quite rightly, it belongs to more than one person.

A well-documented case of the shared paternity of a discovery is that of anaesthetic. It was discovered by two dentists in New England, United States, William Thomas Green Morton (1819–68) and Horace Wells (1815–48), who using the already-known properties of sulphuric ether, "put to sleep" one of their patients in order to painlessly extract their teeth and molars. However, the official date of the discovery was 16 October 1846 when Morton successfully anaesthetised twenty-year-old Gilbert Abbott for an operation on a tumour on his jaw in the great dissection hall of Massachusetts General Hospital in Boston (since then known as the "Ether Dome") by the surgeon John Collins Warren (1778–1856), founder of the famous hospital in 1811.

However, this little tale becomes significantly more complex with the declaration by chemist and geologist Charles Thomas Jackson (1805–80) that he had suggested the ether to Morton, thereby demanding part of the patent. Years later, Crawford Williamson Long (1815–78) would announce that he had been anaesthetising with ether since March of 1842.

Two months after the first famous general anaesthetic in Boston, the British surgeon Robert Liston (1794–1847) would amputate the leg of a patient anaesthetised with ether at the University College Hospital in London.

This saga ends quite tragically with the suicide of Wells in prison and the death of a ruined and bitter Morton some twenty years later.

So we can see that success begets plural paternity, and failure exceptional destitution. On the topic of multiple paternities, the case of penicillin should always be remembered. It was initially discovered in 1929 by Alexander Fleming,* but passed unnoticed for many years until 1941 when it was put to the service of humanity at Oxford University with the work of Howard Florey† and Ernst Boris Chain,‡ (who in 1945 were jointly awarded, justifiably so, the Nobel Prize for Physiology and Medicine. However, public opinion generally only associates the discovery of penicillin with the name Fleming.

Something similar also happened with the discovery of the double helix structure of deoxyribonucleic acid (DNA) by James D. Watson (American, 1928 –) and Francis Crick (British, 1916–2004) at the University of Cambridge, on the one hand, and Maurice Wilkins (of New Zealand origin, 1916–2004) at King's College London, on the other. They were all recognised by the jury of the 1962 Nobel Prize when, as with the case of penicillin, the prize and thereby the corresponding credit for one of the most important scientific discoveries of all time was divided into three equal parts. There was one researcher notably absent, Rosalind Franklin (British, 1920–58, also at King's College London), as she died four years before this exceptional honour was given.

However, it should be stated that in general such fair distribution of

* Alexander Fleming, British microbiologist at St Mary's Hospital in London (1881–1955) † Howard Florey, pathologist of Australian origin
‡ Ernst Boris Chain, chemist of German origin (1906–79)

the corresponding merits is unknown by the general public as it only filters down to certain levels. Sir William Osler (1849–1919) eloquently summed this up when he said: "In science the credit goes to the man who convinces the world, not to the man to whom the idea first occurs." (Osler, cited in Silverman, Murray & Bryan, 2008: 264)

The significance of medicine

To obtain an idea of what medicine of our generation represents, I refer to the authoritative opinion of British historian Arnold Toynbee (1889–1975) who declared:

> The twentieth century will be chiefly remembered by future generations not as an era of political conflicts or technical inventions, but as an age in which human society dared to think of the welfare of the whole human race as a practical objective. (Toynbee cited in Knowles, 1999: 780)

The right to health

This is the concept written into the Venezuelan Constitution, which lays down the fundamental law of Venezuela, in a way that is devoid of all realism. It refers continually, incidentally a bad habit of universal nature, to "*the right to health*", when what they really mean is "*the right to health services or medical services*".

Criticism of medicine

For reasons of space, the "paradoxes" that we have identified are only a simple list accompanied by very brief commentaries designed to outline the nature of the problem. There is no in-depth analysis as the point of these writings is simply to draw the attention of doctors and the general public to the magnitude of the problems that hound the future development of our profession. Many of the statistics used in this work come from the United States, not only because they are reliable or because

English has become the universal *lingua franca*, but because they are continually compared and analysed in multiple published and discussed works, and this facilitates an objective and balanced interpretation of the issues at hand.

A quick flick through the hypercritical books written recently by doctors and laypeople leads us to understand that this is a subject of great, in fact critical, importance for contemporary society, and it would show great astuteness and wisdom on the part of the medical profession to dedicate time to an in-depth study of issues that are no longer their exclusive realm and interest as they become the primary motivation for a universal debate on this sector in public policy material.

I think that the most intelligent and constructive attitude of the medical profession, via its more qualified institutions, would be to give serious attention to the severe, often unjustified, criticisms that have been made recently of contemporary medicine. As the objective of this writing is not to contradict those who have presented a negative image of medicine, I'm limited to providing a list of those publications that I consider most widely available and influential, which I have included as an addendum at the end of this book.

The biologist Sir Peter Medawar (1915–87), winner of the Nobel Prize for Physiology or Medicine (1960), referring to books that he described as "disaffected" and "whining" like that of Ivan Illich* and Thomas McKeown,† wrote the following, which I consider to be a fundamental and very human argument:

"Enjoying the two-fold qualification of being a biologist and having suffered two very grave illnesses I am in a stronger position than either to emphasize the importance of a human being's very strongly marked

* Ivan Illich, Controversial scholar, theologian and philosopher, political and radical social thinker, of Austrian origin (1926–2002)
† Thomas McKeown British doctor, social medical philosopher (1911–88)

26

preference for being alive as opposed to being dead. So long as this preference remains an important element of the human psyche, so long will medical treatment, if necessary of a strenuous and heroic character, remain in demand." (Medawar, 1980)

Other commentators on current medicine try to be more balanced and fair in their evaluations, like the French writer Hervé Hamon (1946–) who publicly declared in his book *Nos Médecins* that he had become interested in doctors because of the crises they are suffering: crisis of identity, economic crisis, ethical crisis, epistemological crisis, and that their crises (that of the doctors) are inevitably our crises (that of all human beings, obviously).

Who can disagree? And, is it not fair perhaps that we doctors ourselves participate in the debate, in order to make our arguments and points of view known?

In these varied critical contributions to medicine there has been no lack of humour, that indispensable stroke of human genius. It is deployed masterfully by a member of the profession in the book *The Alarming History of Medicine* by Doctor Richard Gordon (1921–), author of some forty novels related to medical matters.

The original paradoxes

Three centuries ago in the eighteenth century, the monk and philosopher Spaniard Benito Jerónimo Feijoo (1676–1764) chose the same topic of "Medical Paradoxes" for his work *The Universal Critical Theatre* (Volume Eight, Chapter Ten), in which he said that his books had proposed various medical maxims that "by being contrary to common opinion, can be given the name Paradoxes". (Feijoo, 1726) Father Feijoo cites a similar work by a contemporary of his, Hungarian Miguel Luís Synapio who was seemingly interested in refuting Hippocrates. Feijoo's paradoxes bear no resemblance or similarity to those included in this book, for they are critical, in the most part justifiably so, of the medical practices of his age. He does, however, make a valid conclusion when he declares: "My attempt (for it will be enough if I have even got some things right) is to instil in those doctors who follow the herd a prudent and moderate distrust of received dogmas, because they should never lose sight of the documents of the Master of Medicine, which is experience." (Feijoo, 1726) He also admonishes us with another piece of wise advice: "In order for this warning of never losing sight of the majesty of experience to be useful, it is necessary to add another. Experience doesn't mean a thing if it is not accompanied by shrewd reflection; before proceeding to spread any errors from which one has learned." (Feijoo, 1726)

Definitive Moments in Contemporary Medicine

As described by James Le Fanu* in his book *The Rise and Fall of Modern Medicine* (2011), medicine of the last century has had its "definitive moments". In fact it has had a total of 36 of these moments, listed chronologically below, which represent a good departure point for our analyses. The twelve marked in bold are those he considers to be "definitive":

1935	Sulphonamides
1941	**Penicillin**
	'Pap' smear for cervical cancer
1944	Kidney dialysis
1946	General anaesthesia with curare
1947	Radiotherapy (the linear accelerator)
1948	Intraocular lens implant for cataracts
1949	**Cortisone**
1950	**Smoking identified as the cause of lung cancer**
	Tuberculosis cured with streptomycin and PAS

* James Le Fanu (1950–), British doctor and columnist in the British newspaper *The Daily Telegraph*

1952	The Copenhagen polio epidemic and the birth of intensive care
	Chlorpromazine in the treatment of schizophrenia
1954	The Zeiss operating microscope
1955	**Open heart surgery**
	Polio vaccination
1956	Cardiopulmonary resuscitation
1957	Factor VIII in haemophilia
1959	The Hopkins Endoscope
1960	Oral contraceptive pill
1961	Levodopa for Parkinson's
	Charnley's hip replacement*
1963	**Kidney transplantation**
1964	**Prevention of strokes**
	Coronary bypass graft
1967	First heart transplant
1969	Prenatal diagnosis of Down's Syndrome
1970	Neonatal intensive care
	Cognitive therapy
1971	**Cure of childhood cancer**
1973	CAT scanner
1978	**First test-tube baby**
1979	Coronary angioplasty
1984	**Helicobacter as the cause of peptic ulcer**
1987	Thrombolysis (clot-busting) for heart attacks
1996	Triple therapy for AIDS
1998	Viagra for the treatment of impotence

It is impossible to disagree with Le Fanu in this evaluation of medical progress between 1935 and 1998. It is thanks to these innovations and discoveries that contemporary medicine has gained the prestige that it

---

* Sir John Charnley (1911–82), British orthopedic surgeon, pioneer of hip replacement

enjoys today; a prestige that it must attempt to maintain and increase. If any addition to this list were necessary I would have no hesitation in including the discovery of insulin for the control of diabetes at the University of Toronto in 1922 by Canadian researchers Frederick Grant Banting (1891–1941), Charles Best (1899–1978), James Bertrand Collip* and J. J. R. Macleod (1876–1935); true heralds for this series of discoveries that have completely changed our vision of the world.

Le Fanu also describes what he considers to be the four great paradoxes of modern medicine, three of which are included below.

James Le Fanu's 1st Paradox: Disillusioned doctors
Achievements that were in their time thrilling and emotional (such as the introduction of the pump that replaces cardiac action during heart operations) have come to be matters of mere routine that no longer awaken the same interest. Moreover, due to the fact that admission to medical school has come to be highly competitive, young doctors are much more capable than before and as such less tolerant of the routine of ordinary medical practice.

James Le Fanu's 2nd Paradox: The worried well
This type of public is on the increase, and according to Le Fanu the currently fashionable "social theory" makes them all the more neurotic. The pressure of these healthy people consulting their doctors also coincides with the rising popularity of alternative medicine.

What was previously considered as the practice of medicine men and magicians has become a respectable activity by those who practise homeopathy, naturopathy, acupuncture, etc., whose services are now sought by a third of the adult population.

* James Bertrand Collip (1892–1965) also discovered Adrenocorticotropic hormone

30

James Le Fanu's 4th Paradox: The spiralling costs of health care

The greater the ability of medicine, the higher the demand and consequently the cost.

The growth model is going in the direction of trying to improve the chronic and degenerative illnesses that affect old people. The funds dedicated to this aim, which constitute a weighty proportion of investment in health, have doubled in a decade in the United States, going from 391 billion to 668 billion dollars, without invoking any significant improvement that would justify the scale of the increase.

Author's interpretation

With 62 years of graduate medicine under my belt, and with that particularly intimate relationship with the medical profession that is borne of being surrounded by a family of doctors, what better service could I personally offer to this vocation and passion that I feel so deeply than that of uninhibitedly expressing the anxieties that I feel for the future of this noble job? By expressing my own and other people's concerns, my intention is to correct any possible deviations and open up a debate on the solutions to the many problems we are facing.

In order to give this work a sense of the truly human, I felt it necessary to include some "medical anecdotes", which I have incorporated where they seem best suited to the "paradoxes" being outlined. Some of them have the added value of being humorous, a component that is indispensable and highly healthy in the behaviour of individuals of our species.

Historical unity of medicine

The best proof of the historical unity of the medical profession is represented by the so-called Hippocratic oath, which has established a continuity of ethical behaviour in doctors for over 2,500 years. It is recommended that doctors re-read it once in a while. I copy the text below:

The Hippocratic Oath

I swear by Apollo the physician, and Asclepius, and Hygieia and Panacea and all the gods and goddesses as my witnesses that, according to my ability and judgement, I will keep this Oath and this contract:

To hold him who taught me this art equally dear to me as my parents, to be a partner in life with him, and to fulfil his needs when required;

to look upon his offspring as equals to my own siblings, and to teach them this art, if they shall wish to learn it, without fee or contract; and that by the set of rules, lectures, and every other mode of instruction, I will impart a knowledge of the art to my own sons, and those of my teachers, and to students bound by this contract and having sworn this Oath to the law of medicine, but to no others.

I will use those dietary regimens which will benefit my patients according to my greatest ability and judgement, and I will do no harm or injustice to them.

I will not give a lethal drug to anyone if I am asked, nor will I advise such a place.

Nor will I give a woman a pessary to cause an abortion.

In purity and according to divine law I will carry out my life and my art. I will not use the knife, even upon those suffering from stones, but I will leave this to those who are trained in this craft.

Into whatever homes I go, I will enter them for the benefit of the sick, avoiding any voluntary act of impropriety or corruption, including the seduction of women or men, whether they are free men or slaves.

Whatever I see or hear in the lives of my patients, whether in connection with my professional practice or not, which ought not to be spoken of outside, I will keep secret, as considering all such things to be private. So long as I maintain this Oath faithfully and without corruption, may it be granted to me to partake of life fully and the practice of my art, gaining the respect of all men for all time.

However, should I transgress this Oath and violate it, may the opposite be my fate.

HIPPOCRATES 400 BC[§]

The meaning of humour

To fully understand the importance of paradoxes, and before going into greater detail, I wish to turn to the meaning of humour, for as said by the German writer Dietrich Schwanitz (1940–2004), ". . . humour is part of democracy, for democracy itself rests in a paradox, 'we agree to disagree', and communal harmony is based on permanent discussion. Fanatics and ideologists are panicked by paradoxes; whereas humour is the capacity to put up with insoluble contradictions without losing one's nerve. As long as the dam is raised against the doctrinarians, humour is the democratic attitude *par excellence*". (Schwanitz, 2002)

Fully sharing this view, I have tried to incorporate an element of humour in this essay, whenever I have felt it to be possible, permissible and just.

Human dignity

This is undoubtedly the key factor in fully understanding doctor-patient relationships.

To understand the true meaning of this assertion allow me to

§ *Alfred Kopf, MD: Over the 2500 years or so since the Oath was conceived, things have changed. For example, 'to be partner in life and to fulfill his needs of who taught me this art,' is hardly done today. And 'to look upon his offspring as equals to my own' and 'to teach them this art without fee or contract' must be truly rare today.*

refer to a personal anecdote, which occurred during my capacity as Permanent Delegate, Ambassador of Venezuela to UNESCO in Paris. At that time I was trying to promote the candidacy of Muhammad Yunus (1940–), the creator of the Bank for the Poor, for the Simón Bolívar Prize (which I eventually achieved). One fine day, a Bangladeshi lady turned up at my office dressed in an elegant traditional sari, she had a small office at the UNESCO headquarters and was equally interested in the candidacy of Professor Yunus. The conversation turned towards the meaning of "the bank for the poor" in her country, especially for women, and she told me a moving story. It was about an illiterate woman, with children but no husband, who having heard in her small village about the unsecured loans being offered by this new bank decided to find out if she could seek a loan in order to set up a mini-business in the sale of women's articles (perfumes, costume jewellery, fabric, etc.) at the local market. She thought a sum of as little as one US dollar (its equivalent in rupees) would be sufficient to start her off. The workers at the bank explained to her that it was not possible to give her such a small loan, but that they thought her idea was appropriate and that they would be able to lend her the minimum that the institution was accustomed to. The lady thought about it a while and then rejected the offer and left, claiming that she was uncertain whether she would be able to repay that amount. She subsequently returned to insist on the loan of the original amount she had in mind but was always given the same answer. Eventually one day she accepted the loan and started her business. The idea was an original one as women in Muslim countries were not accustomed to carrying out business in the market. However, very soon the men who visited the market realised that the guidance and advice of a woman were convenient for those looking for a present for their wife, daughter, mother or girlfriend, and for this reason they favoured the lady's business, and

34

she saw her commercial activity prosper quickly. In a short period of time she was able to open other similar businesses in the small villages of the region. The news reached the capital and journalists came to interview this successful woman. She explained to them that her origins were very humble, that in fact before she began the business she was a beggar who lived, together with her youngest children, from the money that she begged on a daily basis. When they asked her about her current economic success she answered without a moment's hesitation that the important thing for her was not the money, but that she had recovered her dignity as a human being. Many people thought that being poor, this woman, and those who shared this extreme poverty, did not know what *dignity* was, however, it is the most deep-rooted and ennobling feeling of the human race. Losing it has an immense moral significance, as this anecdote demonstrates.

It is interesting to note that in his recent book *Health Wars*, the highly qualified critic of current medicine, Doctor Richard Horton (1961–), editor of the famous British weekly medical journal *The Lancet*, has no hesitation in stating that personal health and public health are not "lifestyle" problems but matters of deep existential and geopolitical concern. Reflecting on its implications for our culture, he views medicine as a fractured and rapidly changing discipline, under unprecedented social, political, financial and scientific pressure. But he insists that it must be guided by an ideal above all else: the dignity of the individual facing the illness. His argument for the restoration of dignity is the culmination of an impassioned call to doctors to help structure essential debates on matters from health and curing to the most urgent demands of human development and social justice. (Horton, 2003)

THE GREAT PARADOXES OF CURRENT MEDICINE

1st Paradox
The science of medicine vs. The art of medicine

Medicine is an inseparable and complex mixture of science and art. It has been considered a profession since the ancient times of the father of medicine, Hippocrates of Kos (460–377 BC), although given medicine's theoretical component it could be considered a gratifying and elaborate euphemism for what a profession actually is. The contemporary trend of reducing medicine to an interpretive practice of the most sophisticated technologies, and doctors to mere technologists, thereby limiting and even attempting to undermine their deep "humanism", has created a conflict of incalculable proportions. The negative consequences of this are already visible in a critical decrease in both self-esteem and satisfaction in recently graduated doctors, and in the collective regard for our profession.

The temptation for a destabilising scientific dominance is overwhelming and there is talk, with some justification, of a Holy Grail of medicine: the prevention of those chronic illnesses more prevalent in later life, such as cancer, myocardium, cerebrovascular accidents, Alzheimer's disease, schizophrenia, diabetes and many others, through intervention at a genetic or protein level.

The Genome and Proteomics Eras

At the beginning of this century, the Genome Era gave way to the so-called Proteomics Era, whose champions promised dramatic results both in the short and medium term. They claimed, "people will visit the doctor with their medical histories digitised on plastic cards, similar to the credit cards of today, a kind of marriage between medicine and public health; each card will contain their entire genetic code and medicine will change direction towards a true family medicine, based on the genetics of each family group" – Allen D. Roses.*

The study of medicine

These days, students of medicine cannot limit themselves to studying just anatomy, physiology, embryology, biochemistry, pharmacology and anatomical pathology, as was the case in my student days. Instead they must explore the secrets of cell biology, the molecules inside and outside of cells, the membrane that surrounds the cells, the energy forces that affect them and other related mysteries. "The future of basic medical research is in the hands of geneticists and immunologists and perhaps even psychobiology. In spite of the fact that they have never set foot in a medical laboratory, there are mathematicians, physicists, chemists and engineers who are researching matters that will lead to great advances in the art of curing in the next century."

Futurology is a dangerous discipline and an uncertain intellectual exercise, but these predictions are easy to believe.

Critics of medicine

However, for the French economist, writer and thinker Jacques Attali (1943–), "Soon man won't be a precious machine, a producer of resources, and, thereby, of the facility to cure, but instead a slave to consumerism, and therefore, to production" . . . "In the fog of present day, the crisis in medicine clearly illuminates a future in which curing disappears behind selling, where life and death, the pathological and the normal, the natural and the artificial, become indistinguishable."

* Allen D. Roses, American neurologist from Duke University

Dr Robert S. Mendelsohn*, a self-confessed "medical heretic", makes the case for critics within the medical profession itself: "modern medicine is closer to a religion than to a traditional concept of mixing science and art, as it straddles complex and mysterious matters such as birth, death and all of the tricks that our bodies play on us – and us on them." (Mendelsohn, 1979)

In his book *Human Guinea Pigs*, Maurice Pappworth (1910–94) cites the opinion of Sir William Heneage Ogilvie[†]: "The science of experimental medicine is something new and sinister; for it is capable of destroying in our minds the old faith that we, the doctors, are the servants of the patients whom we have undertaken to care for, and, in the minds of the patients, the complete trust that they can place their lives or the lives of their loved ones in our care." (Ogilvie cited in Pappworth, 1967: 8)

When criticism of the current medical practice, specifically experimentation on humans, comes from a colleague, as in this case, it is perhaps the rule rather than the exception that the medical profession will protest that one of their own is "casting the first stone". This was in fact the case with Pappworth, who paid a high price for his "audacity", suffering true ostracism and other reprisals from the medical profession.

For an observer as perceptive as Sir Peter Medawar, when people talk of the "art and science" of medicine they generally confuse ideas, presuming that the "art" refers to talking to the patient and showing sympathy for them, and the "science" is the more difficult task of interpreting the sophisticated tests to which the patient is submitted in order to reach a diagnosis. According to Medawar, the case is completely the reverse. The true "science" of medicine is the comprehension of its

* Dr Robert S. Mendelsohn (1926–88), North American paediatrician

† Sir William Heneage Ogilvie (1887–1971), Surgeon at Guy's Hospital, London

place in the nature of the medical problem, which is reached by talking extensively with the patient and a physical examination that permits the discovery of any relevant signs of disease. An understanding of the issue will be found in 90% of cases by using this orthodox medical approach. By contrast, many of the more modern technologies, those that pass for "science", are frequently incorrect in their interpretation. The logic of Medawar's argument is based on the paradox that while a doctor may be more reliant on laboratory tests, the medicine that the doctor practises has become less "scientific".

Part of the criticism of medicine, perhaps the most important part, is very common and derives from the same roots that impact on science today. This is summarised by the words of Lewis Wolpert[*] and Alison Richards[†]: "Present attitudes towards science seem to indicate both ambivalence and polarization. While there is much interest and admiration for science, there is also a deep seated fear and hostility. Science is perceived as materialist and dehumanizing, arrogant and dangerous. Its practitioners are a band of cold and unfeeling technicians wielding power without responsibility. Reductionism is suspect and uncomfortable, sabotaging all the mystery and wonder of life. The threats of nuclear war and the genetic manipulation of embryos loom large." (Wolpert & Richards, 1998: 1)

As unjustified or exaggerated as it may seem, as doctors we cannot allow ourselves the luxury of ignoring this type of perception and criticism. We must evaluate such opinions objectively and calmly, and try to correct any misguided conduct that we know to have any basis or foundation.

[*] Lewis Wolpert (1929–), South African biologist who works at University College London
[†] Alison Richards, British scientific journalist

2nd Paradox
Demographic explosion vs. Quality of life

Although a controversial subject, Planet Earth with the seven billion people who inhabit it, geographically at least appears to have reached near saturation levels, especially if we wish to respect and maintain its principal ecological systems.

The worldwide population of our species increased to one billion (a thousand million people) between our first appearance on the planet and the year 1830. A century later, by 1930, the number of inhabitants had doubled to 2 billion; by 1960, to 3 billion; by 1975, to 4 billion; by 1986, to 5 billion; and by 1999 we had crossed the threshold of 6 billion. At the time of writing these lines (February 2014), the estimated population of our planet has already reached 7.2 billion. Unless these figures show signs of levelling off soon, our Earth's bio-sphere will not cope with the stress of this demographic explosion.

At first glance, medicine could be seen as an obvious victim of its own success. Let's look at why. Modern medicine along with hygiene, although perhaps only in a small way, is largely responsible for the recent demographic explosion. Thanks to the advance and progress of medicine, infant mortality has drastically diminished and the average life span of the planet's inhabitants has increased considerably.

At the beginning of the nineteenth century, the infant mortality rate was 250 in every 1,000 births; by 1900 it had dropped to 150 in every 1,000; 10 years later it was 100 in every 1,000 (in fact it was even less than 20 in 1,000 in the last few years of the 1980s). By 2012 the rate had dropped to 7 in every 1,000 in the United States of America.

In Europe at the beginning of the eighteenth century half of children died before they reached the age of 15. Given that a population tends to reach its maximum level of productivity when in its 40s and 50s, this resulted in the loss of important human potential. By 2010 life expectancy had averaged out worldwide to 67.2 years.

This double achievement, spectacular as it has been, has resulted in the negative effects of a demographic explosion that threatens to erode, and at times even destroy, the very environment that should be respected and whose maintenance in balance with the human population that inhabits the planet is essential for the future of the species.

Another factor, with potentially very negative consequences, is that the populations of advanced countries are inclined to stabilise or destabilise, in evident contrast with developing countries whose populations continue to grow in an explosive and worrying manner. In other words, those who have the wealth, capital and technology required to improve conditions of life, have managed to control their demographic growth and with all probability will manage to maintain or increase their quality of existence and pass it on to future generations. By contrast, the world's poor will continue multiplying, making it ever more improbable that they will be able to extract themselves from this vicious circle.[§] Rates of reproduction (the average number of children that every woman has in her life) in countries like Spain, Italy and Japan vary between 1.1 and 1.5, way below the replacement rate which is 2.2.

These figures are concerning because they will cause the continual increase of middle age in those countries; by 2050 this will be 40 in the United States (it was 19 in 1850), 54 in Germany, 56 in Japan and 58 in Italy. It is estimated that half of the populations of developed countries will be at retirement age or older by this date.

§ *Alfred Kopf, MD: "The world's poor will continue multiplying" elicits the question: What is "poor"? As we traveled the world, many people have a high quality of life, even though they lack a lot of resources. They often have a "good" life. What if in future millennia mankind decides to "eliminate" poverty? Look what is happening in China where "poor" is decreasing (as I understand it) in their population of over one billion people.*

Edward O. Wilson* has stood out throughout his teaching and research career as one of the brightest minds on the tortuous and little understood road of the integration of natural sciences and other disciplines, including social sciences, humanities and the arts, in a genuinely titanic effort to obtain "unity of understanding" – an ever complex and difficult process of intellectual synthesis. In his book, *The Future of Life*, he explains to us with measured clarity, that "the ecological footprint" (Wilson, 2002), the average amount of fruitful earth and shallow sea that is attributed to each person from different parts of the world in order to provide them with food, water, habitation, energy, transport, business and absorption of waste, is close to a hectare on average in developed countries, but reaches 9.6 hectares per person in a country with the level of consumption of the United States. If all 7 billion human beings populating the Earth today obtained the scale reached by the North Americans, we would need four planets of the size of ours to cope.

It is highly unlikely that the 3 billion people that make up the developing world will ever reach these high levels, but according to Wilson, if we even come close, it will be sufficient to wipe (that is to say, without human intervention) the last vestiges of natural environment from the face of the planet.

Clearly, medicine cannot be expected, in however small a way, to change its fundamental objectives, which amongst other aspects comprise the two vital parameters already mentioned; its successes in diminishing infant mortality and the lengthening of human life through the cure or controlling of a myriad of illnesses. Viewed from another angle and from a global perspective, this achievement is, for the most part, responsible for one of the largest problems confronted by humanity, that explosive, and as yet uncontrolled, demographic growth in the world's poorest and most in need countries.

* Edward O. Wilson (1929–), Harvard professor, originally from Britain

As Wilson maintains: "At the same time, *Homo sapiens* has become a geographical force, the first species in the history of the planet to attain that dubious distinction. We have driven atmospheric carbon dioxide to the highest levels in at least two hundred thousand years, unbalanced the nitrogen cycle, and contributed to a global warming that will ultimately be bad news everywhere." (Wilson, 2002: 23)

It should also be said that we have invented weapons of mass destruction, atomic and hydrogen bombs, theoretically capable of wiping all traces of life from the surface of the planet (that soft layer that covers the Earth, known as its biosphere); a self-destructive power, with the capacity for total genocide acquired by our species for the first time in history in the mid-twentieth century, the employment of which has so far been avoided through the use of reason amongst those who possess and monopolise this lethal power, a power that is as horrifying as it is threatening.

In other words, whilst its very nature and its success rates are partly the cause of the problem, there is no real possibility that medicine will be able to change current trends. Efforts to level out the current global population escape medicine's capabilities and obey instead the multiple causes that fall outside its powers.

The words of British doctor, Vernon Coleman (1946–), support my view. In the prologue of his book on the future that awaits us he doesn't hesitate to say: "By the year 2020 one third of the population in the developed world will be over the age of 65. One quarter of the population will be diabetic. In every home where there are two healthy parents and two healthy children there will be four disabled or dependent individuals needing constant care. Diseases such as diabetes and schizophrenia (which are genetically transmitted) and blindness (which is ten times as common among the over-65s and 30 times as common among the over-75s) will be as common as indigestion and

45

hayfever are today. Unemployment will be normal. Stress-related diseases will be endemic. Developed countries around the world will face bankruptcy as they struggle to find the cash to pay pensions, sick pay and unemployment benefits . . . The human race will be destroyed by medical ambition, commercial greed, and political opportunism." (Coleman, 1989: 1)

This could be an excessively pessimistic, perhaps even catastrophic and alarmist, view of the future that awaits us, but if we don't urgently change our approach to the problems we are facing, these predictions and their terrible consequences will be unavoidable.

Julio Pérez Díaz* points out: "Humanity is going through a reproductive revolution that allows it, for the first time in history, to reduce fertility (the number of children per woman). This is due to the recently born having a longer life ahead of them than their ancestors . . . It will result in an unprecedented change in the civilisation ahead of them. Its political, economic and social consequences are enormous."

However, I think that the responsibility of doctors in such delicate matters is subordinate to the public's comprehension of the magnitude of the problem. They rely on being informed and educated about current reality by the political classes (and above all by the statistics held by said political classes), in order to bring about public policies that attempt to correct the anomalies introduced by our technological success. By not "taking the bull by the horns" and moving forward with the successful advancement of this process of collective education, we are in danger of bringing about a sort of self-inflicted collective holocaust.

The collective influence that doctors have on society is precisely

* Julio Pérez Díaz (1960–), Spanish demographist and sociologist, who, along with John MacInnes (Scottish sociologist), developed the Theory of the Reproductive Revolution

46

the reason why they can assist with this huge and inevitable task that simply must take priority in the future.

In 1979, after various attempts to control its demographic growth, China – which with its 1.351 billion inhabitants (in 2012) is the most populated country in the world – adopted the tough and controversial decision to permit only one child per family; a policy made possible by their totalitarian communist regime. This policy was maintained until 2013 when they announced the possibility of increasing the "quota" to two children per family, undoubtedly concerned by the effects of an ageing population incapable of achieving predetermined economic goals. One of the many effects of this policy is that currently there are one million parents and grandparents with just a single descendant; undoubtedly influenced by the Confucian philosophy so prevalent in Chinese society, these parents and grandparents are willing to make great economic sacrifices to provide their children with the very best education available. This could be an important factor in the results of the PISA* exam where young people from the province of Shanghai achieve the best results in the world in mathematics, the sciences and language comprehension.

It should be stressed that the great problem remains, those countries capable of successfully managing an overflowing population are the affluent countries of the so-called developed world, whilst as a general rule those that have the highest rates of reproduction are the poorest nations. This takes us in the wrong direction and creates problems that are very hard to resolve. It is clear that the answer in the medium and long term is closely linked to educating women, who in developed countries have taken control of their fertility.

* PISA: established by the OECD, PISA (Programme for International Student Assessment) takes place every three years, with 15-year-olds from 65 nations participating

3rd Paradox
Vegetative life vs. Euthanasia

The dramatic increase in the global population's average lifespan continually threatens to create societies of the elderly, of retirees and pensioners, who will shortly outnumber those people capable of working and producing. This is especially the case in the developed world as the increase in average lifespan is proportionally higher in industrialised, affluent countries with better medical services. All actuarial calculations regarding this matter are out of date and the economic imbalances that they create are a permanent headache for statisticians, and even politicians, worldwide.

However, the essential medical problem is that whilst advances in transplants and other methods have had some success in prolonging the active life of many organs (such as the cornea, the kidney, the heart, the liver, and even the lungs), it is currently impossible, and in all likelihood will continue to be for many years, to do the same with the brain. Some time ago I wrote an article on "the impossible transplant" referring to this very fact, and the mistaken assumption that we could undertake the surgery required to transplant a whole brain into a human body, when what would actually happen would be the transplant of a body to a brain (and not the contrary). This is because what ultimately truly defines the human being is consciousness and the cognitive activity that originates in the brain.

On the other hand, with the increase in the average lifespan, the reasonably effective and acceptable medical and surgical solutions that are being found for problems that develop from the gradual deterioration and erosion of the human body caused by the ageing process and the decreased functionality of organs, tissues, apparatus and systems, bear no relation to the limited advances associated with degenerative diseases of the central nervous system.

Diseases like Alzheimer's, practically unknown five decades ago, are on the steady increase in direct proportional relation to the increase in the average lifespan of populations, and are wreaking havoc in developed countries, leading as they do to a population with a substantial number of old people condemned to a vegetative life. Alzheimer's disease is already accepted as the third cause of death in the United States, after heart disease and cancer. It has become the greatest threat of the future, and a focus of concern for countries like the United States and Great Britain, as it not only incapacitates those who suffer from it, but also creates a need for constant human assistance as the disease progresses, a situation that can carry on for several years, representing very high costs.

Given these circumstances, euthanasia is presented, with considerable social pressure, as a valid solution. It is slowly but surely penetrating the consciousness of traditionally liberal societies such as the Netherlands, where we observe the emergence of the use of euthanasia to put an end to the vegetative life of those old people condemned to this inhuman situation, which eliminates all quality of life.

The steady rise in the length of human life in affluent countries is creating problems for which orthodox Christian morality (especially Catholic morality), so rigid in its views of the sacredness of life, does not yet have appropriate answers.

Transplants make it possible to keep vital organs working, organs like the kidney, the liver or the heart, especially with the use of drugs, like Cyclosporine, that prevent the phenomenon of rejection. However, for all of the state of the art technology that prolongs the life of people who until a generation ago were terminally ill due to vital organ failure, there have not been similar advances as far as a well-performing brain is concerned; the organ on which our consciousness and capacity for reason depend, and which holds the essential component of our humanity.

This is the justification and reasoning of the universal cry of those people who aspire to "die with dignity", who know that "they can demand it as a right". (Betancourt in *El Pais*, 2003)

And so a new human right emerges, the right to die, at least in the eyes of The World Federation of Right to Die Societies.* A right contemplated by the penologist Luis de Jiménez de Asúa (1889–1970) in his book *Libertad de amar y derecho a morir* (The Freedom to Love and the Right to Die) in 1928.

This in other words is a clear acceptance of euthanasia. According to information published by the Centro de Investigaciones Sociológicas (Centre for Sociological Research or CIS) in Spain, 6 out of 10 doctors would support a change in the law "in order to permit ill people to ask for and receive assisted suicide from a doctor and / or active euthanasia".

Furthermore, a survey by the *Organización de Consumidores y Usarios – OCU* (Organisation of Consumers and Users in Spain) states that 70% of Spaniards would like euthanasia to be legalised.§

Euthanasia is already legal in Holland and Belgium and it is said that the pro-euthanasia movement is advancing rapidly in France, Japan and Australia. In Switzerland, the organisation Dignitas offers "assisted suicides" to "those Europeans who wish to use their services".

For the medical profession it is an undoubtedly thorny and difficult issue, as they are viewed by the public, and self-identify, as an institution

---

* The World Federation of Right to Die Societies was established in Oxford in 1980 and now has more than 800,000 members in 27 countries

§ *Alfred Kopf, MD: Should there be the possibility to choose euthanasia rather than "incarceration for life"? To be imprisoned for life to some people is devastating and "not worth living." Furthermore, it is costly to incarcerate for life. Could euthanasia one day become a choice?*

intended to fight for life and combat those illnesses that threaten life. Indeed, the fact that the extension of the lifespan of entire nations has reached, even exceeds, 80 years can in the main part undoubtedly be attributed to medicine. But the price to pay is high, and doubts and anxieties about how to mitigate the negative consequences of a population that is ageing before our eyes are emerging.

Contrary to centuries-old tradition, will it be the medical profession who, at the request of their own patients, put an end to the days of the people they helped bring into the world? It is a cruel question mark that hangs like Damocles' Sword over those who practise this noble profession, and who until now had not needed to seriously consider this highly macabre, sad and desolate proposition.

Perhaps, as my medic son suggests, if this possibility becomes a reality in the future, it should be other professionals, not doctors, who are tasked with the grim procedure, playing not exactly the role of an executioner, but certainly something similar.

4th Paradox
Economic weakness or need vs. Quality of medical attention

Medicine has of old striven to look beyond the racial, religious and cultural prejudice of human beings, and tried via the resources at its disposal to ensure that the economic differences between human beings don't negatively affect those who do not have the necessary means to supply and pay for the medical care they receive; the Hippocratic Oath is in fact established on this basis.

This ideal, which always falls short and is perhaps unattainable, has become more difficult to achieve with every day that passes. New medical technologies, which are more sophisticated and complex than ever, are exceedingly costly; the same can be said of the price of new medicines (as is the case with the patented drugs necessary to maintain the lives of AIDs patients). The gap that exists between the quality of medical services available to those with economic means and those lacking them is wider every day, and dangerously distorts the ethical foundations of the medical profession at a worldwide level. In many countries, adequate medical services are only available to those who can pay for them. Our generation's medical profession has had to accept the draconian rules imposed by the administration of the institutions with which they are affiliated, which may mean that in order to survive they do not have the luxury of offering charity by absorbing the costs of the modern and efficient diagnostic and therapeutic technologies.

When I began my private practice in 1954, the custom in Venezuela, most certainly copied from France where nearly all of my medical teachers specialised, was to dedicate mornings to teaching and working in public hospitals for a nominal salary, and afternoons to private professional practice, where the resources required to maintain a decent level of life and keep a family were truly earned. This was changing progressively at the time and is now possibly the exception rather than the rule.

I discussed this issue in more detail in 1998 at a meeting called "Aula Magna" at the Pontificia Universidad Católica in Peru, published in the book *Ética e Investigación: ¿el fin justifica los medios?* (Ethics and Research: does the end justify the means?), edited by Liliana Regalado de Hurtado and Carlos A. Chávez Rodríguez.

5th Paradox
Lies vs. State secrets

Can lies and the falsification of medical fact in the context of "state secrets" ever be justified?

History has provided many cases of illness in Heads of State, and the problems caused by such cases have been the subject of much study. The methods systematically employed by political and governmental systems to deceive the public clearly demonstrate their creativity and capacity for collusion, more often than not through the collaboration (complicity perhaps?) of the treating physicians.

We have nearly always found out *a posteriori* about the dramas that have taken place within the close administrations of heads of state in order to deliberately hide their true health from the public. In this club, dominated by gerontocracy, it is not unusual that incidences of ill-health amongst these characters are the rule rather than the exception. Many of these problems mentally incapacitate the ill person, in our case the Head of State, from the ability to evaluate their own health (especially if the problem is cerebral), for which reason it would be impractical and naïve to leave the decision in the hands of the patient him or herself. In these cases the treating physician's ethical commitment to the truth is required, disregarding the political pressure that justifies itself in "state secrets".

Recent history offers abundant evidence of a systematic hiding of the truth by authorities in accordance with the complacency, and very often active collaboration, of the doctors responsible.

We can recall the case of Antonio de Oliveira Salazar (1889–1970), dictator of Portugal, who suffered a cerebral thrombosis in 1968; the case of Francisco Franco (1892–1975) who was kept alive for a month using all different kinds of medical resources (including a blood transfusion of more than 50 litres of blood, Franco was tested, dialyzed and refrigerated and kept alive thanks to the continuous work of "indefatigable machines"); the case of Mao Tse-tung (1893–1976) in China, who suffered from progressive arteriosclerosis for ten years and was confined to his palace from 1974; the case of Josip Tito (1892–1980) in Yugoslavia; the case of Leonid Brezhnev (1906–82), the case of Yuri Andropov (1914–84) and Konstantin Chernenko (1911–85) in Soviet Russia, to name but a few dictators; in these cases it was easy to hide the truth and deliberately deceive their citizens using the repressive apparatus of their respective governments.

However, the manipulation of truth for political ends is not just limited to authoritarian regimes. This was revealed recently when Claude Gubler (1934–), doctor to François Mitterrand (1916–96) for many years, published his scandalous book containing details of the ex-president of France's medical history. The publication caused bitter controversy in France and even led to a prison sentence for its author. Shortly after being elected for his first term as President of the Republic of France, Mitterrand discovered that he had prostate cancer with bone metastases. In spite of this, thanks to a variety of treatments, he was able to govern two consecutive presidential terms (14 years), without the public learning of his medical problems. He was able to hand his job over to his successor and even chose the date of his death when he voluntarily suspended the treatment he was undergoing. The doctor (who had distanced himself from his illustrious patient some time before) was found guilty by the Medical Council of France for the publication of a book that was clearly in violation of medical confidentiality, but bizarrely he was not judged on the evident manipulation of the truth, which was consistently adulterated and falsified in annual reports on the health of the President, conveniently protected by state secrets. If we accept that under the mantle of state secrets it is legally and morally possible to manipulate and adulterate medical truth, and that none of the bulletins or communications make any sense as they have been "cooked" in the interests of the politician in office from the outset, of what value and importance are they to the public? It is curious that it is this aspect to which least importance is attributed in the public debate of such a delicate matter.

The case of President Mitterrand was only of relative importance given that his health problems, although bothersome, did not affect his mental capacity, his dedication or his behaviour as Head of State. But what would have happened if the limiting and problematic illness had stemmed from the brain? For how long would his political team have been able to hide the truth from the public? Which and how many decisions would have been made by people who were neither qualified nor legally authorised under the pretence that they were made by the person chosen by the electorate for a position that cannot be delegated and much less carried out by people selected in secret and behind their backs?

Who could have imagined that only a few years later we would experience the same problem in Venezuela with the illness and death of Hugo Chávez Frías (1954–2013)? This case had the added complication that his doctors were all Cuban with his treatments carried out in Cuba, and so it was difficult to determine whether the interests of the supposed state secret were on the Venezuelan or Cuban side. At the time of writing these lines it is still impossible to determine accurately what really happened, but it is possible to say without a shadow of doubt that the truth about the diagnosis and treatment of the President's illness was kept from the Venezuelan public for a long time, a truth manipulated and adulterated by another country in accordance with its own interests.

6th Paradox
Consuming alcohol vs. Good health

Until a few years ago, the medical orthodoxy viewed drinking alcohol as a damaging habit, potentially dangerous in causing addiction in some people, and therefore an unpleasantness that should only be moderately tolerated in order to facilitate social interaction.

However, recent clinical studies on significant sample groups appear irrefutably to demonstrate that daily ingestion of moderate quantities of alcohol is beneficial for your health. In the case of red wine the benefit is attributed to Resveratrol (a phytoalexin found in grapes), an anti-oxidant that prolongs life in test animals.

In truth it is not hard for doctors to reason that the dose can be the difference between benefit and harm, and that the key word in the consumption of alcohol, as in many other cases, is moderation.

For the general public, the distinction is not as simple or direct. Anti-alcoholism health education campaigns are becoming more complex, as given the information in existence it is not possible to absolutely condemn the consumption of alcohol. Certainly, the danger that a small percentage of those who consume alcohol could become addicts is a proven risk that we cannot ignore. Alcoholism is a fairly common disease, exceptionally degrading, difficult to treat and with very negative social consequences for the alcoholic and their family.

The initial hypothesis that lower incidences of cardiovascular illness occur in those who regularly drink moderate amounts of red wine was replaced at a later date, and supported by numerous studies in various countries, by the belief that the beneficial effect was due to alcohol generically (in its diverse forms, whether beer, wine or distilled spirits).

It has been established reasonably well, (one study looked at nearly half a million people over a period of nine years), that drinkers have a 20 –30% lower chance of premature death from cardiovascular illness than those who abstain from alcohol.

The knowledgeable recommend a "drink" a day for women and two "drinks" a day for men (one drink = 12 ounces = 355 ml of beer; or 5 ounces = 148 ml of wine; or 1.5 ounces = 44 ml distilled spirit)

The British health authorities issued guidelines in 1995 establishing that people who don't drink or drink very little in the age group considered at high risk of cardiac illness should "consider the possibility" that ingesting alcoholic drinks in moderate quantities can have health benefits.

In the United States, the American Health Association is more conservative, establishing that if one must drink, it should be with moderation, and that the incidences of heart disease in those that consume moderate quantities of alcohol are lower than in those that abstain, whilst always insisting on the dangers of the consumption of alcohol, such as alcoholism, high blood pressure, obesity, ictus, suicide and accidents. The daily consumption of alcohol can cause severe damage to cardiac muscle fibres (alcoholic myocarditis) and brain cells.

7th Paradox
Organ donation vs. Sale of organs for transplant

A blood transfusion can be considered a tissue (blood) transplant. In many countries there is a tradition of the sale of blood to blood banks by donors who make money from it, for example in the United States.

Fortunately in Venezuela the sale of human blood is not permitted, therefore certain human body parts are excluded from sale for transplant (unlike double organs such as kidneys or bones), other transplantable organs such as the heart require a body to function for they are unique organs and indispensable to the life of the individual.

Within the Christian tradition the two patron saints of doctors (along with Saint Luke), Saint Cosmas and Saint Damian (d. *c.* 287), twin brothers who lived in the Near West at the beginning of our era, carried out (one as anaesthetist, the other as surgeon) the transplant of the leg of a recently deceased black slave to a white patient whose lower leg had been amputated. This was their first miracle, depicted in great paintings in famous museums (one of which we chose for the cover of this book). Nearly two millennia later, Alexis Carrel* would take a colossal technological step with a pair of dogs (one white and one black) when he transplanted a paw from one animal to the other. Many decades later he achieved a hand transplant from a corpse to an accidental amputee. With the help of powerful drugs to impede the rejection of tissues that didn't belong to the body receiving the transplant, what was previously considered a "miracle" soon became a reality of modern surgical technology.

But what should be highlighted here is that contemporary society

* Alexis Carrel, 1873–1944, medical doctor, biologist and writer of French origin and winner of the Nobel Prize for Medicine in 1912, who worked at the Rockefeller Institute for Medical Research in New York

considers the sale of organs immoral and illegal, therefore whoever needs one, and it can often be the difference between life and death, has to find a voluntary and free donor (generally a close family member).

This situation has resulted in the illegal sale of organs by people from developing countries who in return for desperately needed money have no hesitation in depriving themselves of a double organ (generally kidneys) via a delicate surgical procedure.

In some Latin American countries classified adverts are published in newspapers offering kidneys, corneas, etc. for sale. Without a shadow of doubt, the sale of organs exists.

Some time ago I heard a programme on the radio by the BBC in London on reports by various voluntary organisations linking the disappearance of hundreds of women in Mexico to crimes related to the sale of organs. To all appearances, this is a serious problem that we cannot put to one side without an investigation into the source of the concerns raised. The gravity of the case is that in order for a business of such a nature to even be possible, a chain of complicities is needed; complicities that are hard even to imagine.

8th Paradox
Staying in one's country of origin vs. Emigration

Large migrations have always been determined by political circumstances (such as persecutions) or economic circumstances (especially famine), leaving those who are obliged to take this hard road with little choice.

A well-trained doctor, especially if they have already specialised, is of great value to their country of origin (as much for their lengthy training as for its intrinsic value), so losing this human capital, in the case that they do decide to emigrate, represents a great loss for the "donor" country and, by contrast, a win for the "receiving" country.

The cost of training a doctor and the value they represent to the country to which they emigrate was the subject I chose for my incorporation as Honorary Member of the National Academy of Medicine in Colombia in February of 1999. Given the elevated number of Colombian doctors who have emigrated to the United States I thought it would be an interesting subject to initiate a debate, as in some way there is perhaps an element of justice involved as this single contribution would more than compensate for the aid which Colombia, in one capacity or another, has received from the big country to the North (excluding military support against guerrillas and narcotrafficking).

The huge emigration seen in Venezuela in the last 15 years (1999–2013), estimated between 800,000 and 1,000,000 people, is perhaps an unprecedented phenomenon as much for its magnitude (from a country of 30 million inhabitants), as for its quality consisting principally as it does of young university graduates. This is a new problem for a country that until then had experienced rapid population growth due in large part due to the immigration of significant contingents of Italians, Spanish and Portuguese looking for better economic conditions following the Second World War. This country is currently being affected by the opposite phenomenon of losing its trained human resources and, rather explosively, its replacement generation. Although there are surely multiple causes, amongst them deficient remuneration, rejection of the communist ideal, absence of acknowledgement of merit, etc., there is no doubt that the insecurity and impunity permitted and perhaps even sponsored by the current Government are the common denominators in such a difficult and traumatic decision.

The Venezuelan talent abroad programme (TALVEN) is an answer to this migratory problem that has become serious in the last fifteen years.

It is estimated that in the last decade around 7, 100 doctors have emigrated from Venezuela, the majority of them to Spain and the United States. Spain welcomes the arrival of our doctors as it is suffering the same phenomenon with its doctors emmigrating to other European countries (especially Great Britain and Germany) where they are better paid. The Venezuelan medical profession has been compromised by the current regime and suffers the humiliation of seeing its field invaded by supposed doctors from Cuba, who are free to practise medicine without having to revalidate their knowledge as required by the law.

9th Paradox
Family doctors vs. Specialists

Economically speaking there is disproportionate added value between the services of a general practitioner and a specialist doctor.

The training of a specialist is longer and more costly, therefore their time is more economically valuable. In the British health system every patient wishing to see a specialist must first be examined by a General Practitioner (GP) as access to a specialist is not possible without their referral. If we accept as true the statistic that 80% of people who visit a doctor don't require treatment, we understand the incongruity of the matter especially given that we also know that 80% of people who go to see a doctor will receive some form of treatment (although it may not be necessary). I have heard it said several times that when the general public visit a doctor in France they feel cheated if the consultation doesn't end with three different medical prescriptions (hence perhaps the increase in medicines based on exotic herbs with supposed pharmacological effects of doubtful proven scientific foundation, and hence the lenience and complacency of a health authority that is willing to gratify a highly sensitive collective sentiment).

When a sovereign state recognises its responsibility for its population's medical attention it has to understand from the start that the family doctor is the backbone of collective healthcare, and it must therefore use mechanisms and incentives of the most diverse kind to boost this type of training amongst doctors who have recently graduated from university.

10th Paradox
The right to health vs. The right to medical attention

Politicians rule the world, albeit on the basis of false promises, exaggerations and hyperbole. We have become accustomed to hearing them repeatedly talk, without determinable consequences, about an infinity of "human rights", such as the rights of children, of homosexuals, right to life, right to death, rights of the accused, rights of criminals (we know of institutions and people dedicated to this sole purpose), rights of victims (a little more logical and socially acceptable than the previous one), right to periodic holidays, even the rights of animals, and why not, perhaps one day even plants will have rights.

Even within this veritable jungle of all types of rights (rarely accompanied by their corresponding "duties" as ought to occur in a just and balanced "social contract"), it is odd, entertaining, and even a little ridiculous to see how the constituents are devoted to Article 83 of our brand-new "Bolivarian Constitution", the most modern and "revolutionary" of all the constitutions. This outlines the so-called "right to health", which is defined as follows: "Health is a fundamental social right, an obligation of the State, who will guarantee it as part of the right to life." Therefore, this is a right that the Venezuelan state should supposedly guarantee to all of its citizens, but it so happens that neither this State nor other more advanced States for that matter are able to guarantee the health of all of its citizens. They are not, nor will they ever be capable of doing so, because quite simply it doesn't depend on them, rather on multiple factors that they don't control nor will they be able to control in the foreseeable future. For example and without going any further, the degenerative diseases caused by ageing and the erosion of the human body, which the future advance of medicine can perhaps defer for a few years but will never be able to postpone indefinitely or manage to eradicate.

64

But nobody raises his or her voice to decry the politicians' latest deceit (and not only Venezuelan politicians if we are going to be fair), which is nothing more than an easily proven hypocrisy. If this so-called "right to health" were at least changed, manipulated and "sweetened" to something less unequivocal, ambitious and pompous, like for example, "the right to medical attention", perhaps it would be more digestible, realistic and acceptable. It would at least demonstrate the unavoidable duty of the State to ensure the ideal, and let's be clear about what an ideal is – it is something quite intangible – to aspire and contribute to the good health of its citizens, calling on medical services, amongst other means, which should be subsidised by the government for the poor who lack the funds to cover medical costs. We would at least have no inhibitions in recognising the good intention that guided legislators in aspiring to an ideal that infrequently and with much effort, is achieved in very few affluent, cultured and well-administrated nations. But establishing constitutionally and in the most dogmatic and forceful way that the Venezuelan State "guarantees" to all of its citizens the "right to health", that is to say, a right on which they can exercise only a relative influence, is nothing more than another nonsensicality, one more ridiculous thing, one more absurdity, of the many to which we are unhappily accustomed.

11th Paradox
Fair fees vs. Abusive fees

As medical fees are generally based on the quality of the expertise and the time spent with each patient, there are no well-defined rules that indicate their value. However, in recent decades medical insurance companies have become involved to such a degree that they set the fees for many surgical or medical procedures, thereby establishing the parameters that determine professional fees, which therefore vary from country to country, and even from town to town.

Unlike other white-collar professions that deal in business matters, who are able to value their fees according to how much they trade, doctors must, to a certain degree, look beyond the personal finances of the patient (which are generally ignored and not referred to during the consultation). This is perhaps a little unfair as any failure in the care of an affluent or famous patient can result in seriously negative economic consequences for the doctor, when often what is at stake is the prosperous patient's life.

The fact is that a sick person is so worried and nervous about the eventual outcome of their illness that they tend to think that any sum of money is small when their health is at stake, yet as soon as they recover, their way of thinking changes. Let us recall the anecdote attributed to the famous British surgeon Lord Lister (1827–1912), who was required to attend to a rich nobleman who had a fishbone stuck in his throat. The great surgeon removed the fishbone with considerable skill. Grateful for his efficient attention, the patient asked Lister for his fee. Lister smiled pleasantly and replied: "My Lord, suppose we settle for half of what you would be willing to give me if the bone were still lodged in your throat." (V. K. Subramanian, 2004: 93)

Plastic and reconstructive surgery, a specialism that was nobly born to attend to and repair the deformities and mutilations of soldiers who fought in the First World War has, little by little, at least in large part, turned into a surgery of embellishment; a battle, scalpel in hand, against the ravages of old age on the human body.

Plastic surgery, inflated as it presently is by consumerist public demand both in affluent countries and also in the economically privileged sectors of poorer countries, deals with, sometimes exclusively, aesthetic problems born of human vanity. As far as professional fees are concerned, it is not governed by any parameters or rates, as these are clearly elective procedures that do not bear any relation to the health of a person. The fees are therefore based on other criteria such as the reputation of the professional or the socioeconomic importance of the patient, for which reason the variations are extreme and very often inexplicable even according to market forces. Consequently, this type of surgery particularly lends itself to fees that are disproportionate to the procedure being carried out and exposes the medical profession, by unjustified generalisation, to discredit and acid judgement.

12th Paradox
Doctors vs. Lawyers

It is said that in a society where there are more lawyers than doctors (like North American society, where the ratio is approximately 2.5:1), there are undoubtedly distortions in which litigant elements overflow and invade all the areas habitually reserved for the good judgement and discretion of the doctor, whose competence and honour in previous eras were taken for granted. After all, who feeds the lawyers, if they don't continually create legal problems to which they must attend?

Whilst the issue is not provoked by one simple cause alone, such as the numerical relation of lawyers to doctors in practice in a given country, it is an important element to consider.

On the other hand, it is impossible to deny that medical practice undertaken without due preparation or with a lack of up-to-date information can negatively affect the health of patients (iatrogenic illnesses), which can in turn be a significant cause of illness.

This has led to a vicious circle that has notably contributed to an increase in medical costs. Doctors are obliged to pay high insurance premiums for their "malpractice" cover, the cost of which, like it or not, must pass as soon as possible to the patient, by discreetly including it in their bill. At the end of the day, it is the patient who ends up paying these increased costs, either directly, or via an increase in premiums for those who are insured.

In 1971, between 12,000 and 15,000 professional malpractice lawsuits were presented in the courts of the United States. Less than half of these lawsuits were resolved within 18 months, and more than 10% remained unresolved for more than 6 years. For every dollar paid in professional malpractice insurance, 16 to 20 cents goes to compensating the victim; the rest is paid to the lawyers and medical experts.

At my request, the lawyer, and my good friend, Juan Francisco Lloán, wrote the commentary below:

It is not so simple. After 1945, in the United States, as in the whole of the West, there was a disillusionment, an inhibition, a complex, about what the Law ought to be (the axiological aspect), that it ought to concentrate on the being (positivism): the Law is what is written, everything else would be behind it: culture, tradition, values (perish the thought!), the sense of common good that would arise from the awareness of a shared future: all of this has been thrown out. Through cowardice, abandoning principles, and intimidation. Only the bold Orwellian discourse of the social-ists, as "fools rush in where angels fear to tread", has imposed "socialists reasons" that oust the positive Law. It has inevitably resulted in a legal practice that is interpreted in a utilitarian and, inevitably, for that reason financial sense. The widespread loss of values has removed any shame from greed. Hence the spread of pirate trials. Moreover, this, of course, has clearly not escaped medicine. So, in a way, American society, where the traditional tendency is for legal disputes (A. de Tocqueville *dixit*), has degenerated into a deluge of real or supposed "malpractice" claims, and the consequent necessary economic distortion of the large insurance covers required for professional practice. I recall that before this was the fashion, there was already a proliferation of peculiar claims: i.e. the claim against the producer of a floor wax that caused the victim to slip; against the barman who serves too many drinks to the person who later drives and kills somebody, etc. Let me finish with a Jewish joke: asked why Israel always won the wars started by its neighbours, the Israeli commander cryptically said: "Oh we just put our lawyers and doctors on the front line, and we order them "CHARGE!!!" . . . (Pause) . . . and you know how the bastards charge!" On the other hand, it is unfortunately true that the victims asking for compensation generally end up receiving only a small part of the "award" from the courts (or from the transaction that generally, in the majority of cases, puts an end to the case). This last situation would call for corrective legislation of a federal nature.

13th Paradox
Reproductive medicine vs. Reproductive manipulation

The reproductive medicine sector is one of the most advanced of the recent past. It contributes efficiently to resolving many of the problems faced by infertile couples who in previous generations did not have the technological solutions of modern medicine at their disposal.

These advances have revealed a series of initially unforeseen uses, and sometimes abuses, that question head-on the very moral basis of contemporary society, which, after considerable consideration, will undoubtedly have to change in order to adapt to this new knowledge, as has happened consistently in the past. As with the case of human cloning, this has led to an intense, bitter and ferocious debate.

Given the technological advances already achieved, the possibilities of undesirable manipulations of reproductive material are infinite. Three examples suffice to illustrate this point:

A few years ago, a newspaper from the West coast of the United States published a report on a North American millionaire couple, each with children from their first marriages. During a visit to Australia, they left some of the wife's fertilised ovaries (eggs or zygotes) frozen in a local institution. Many years later, the husband having died, the widow conceived a child using one of the eggs. It's easy to imagine the mess that this caused, the legal chaos of a child born five years after the death of his or her father and the problems engendered by the sharing of inheritance, etc. As it turns out, the reporter invented the story, but the problems that could potentially occur are real, this is not science fiction but a real possibility in this new reality of in vitro fertilisation.

Then there's the doctor from the south of the United States who artificially inseminated a large number of female patients with his own spermatozoa. By the time this criminal outrage was revealed, the fertility specialist had nearly as many "biological" children as General Juan Vicente Gomez.* What legal avenue should be recommended to these mothers to punish the crime of the "biological" father of their children? How should these children view their "biological" father?

Finally, the story published in a weekly newspaper of worldwide circulation (accompanied by full colour photographs), told the well-documented tale of the Dutch lady, married to a Dutchman (both Caucasian), who after treatment at a fertility clinic in her country gave birth to twins, one black and one white. The subsequent investigation revealed that there had been some confusion at the lab and that the semen of a patient from the Dutch Antilles had accidentally penetrated one of the lady's ovaries, whilst the other was fertilised by her husband's spermatozoa.

* General Juan Vicente Gomez (1857–1935), was the dictator of Venezuela from 1908 until his death in 1935. He kept a written record of the names of his 74 children

14th Paradox
Employees vs. Administrators

Within the service sector medical attention has possibly lagged behind those rules that dictate the market economy, perhaps due to that unavoidable and quite particular relationship between patient and doctor. However, the trend in industrialised countries is very clear, and doctors in the practice of their liberal profession are more and more subject to the regulations and impositions of the largest industry in the world, that is to say the health industry, which is governed by rules that are completely different to those to which doctors were accustomed a mere generation ago.

In essence, doctors have become the employees, and in some cases administrators, of just one more business; the business of the health of people or even entire populations.

Doctors have to learn to interact with hospital administrators, who generally aren't doctors and so only partially understand the values and principles of medical deontology. They must negotiate with these people who are essentially looking after the interests of a business, even though they may call it a clinic or a hospital. They must also consider the rights and duties of patients, doctors and other health personnel, the rights of the employees and of the financial institution to which they owe their principal loyalty and institutional dependency, and ultimately on whose economic solvency they all depend.[§]

It is clear that this is a new and complex situation in which the medical profession must intelligently and creatively intervene.

§ *Alfred Kopf, MD: Many physicians in the USA are quitting private practice and retiring prematurely or joining medical groups/hospital staffs full time to avoid the burdensome rules and regulations imposed by so many organizations (mostly government, and even their own medical societies imposing Continuing Medical Education tests). Many doctors prefer seeing patients to filling out more and more forms.*

15th Paradox
The medical act: Complete vs. Partial

The ideal of course is for one person only to be responsible for the whole medical experience, as when actions are divided so too are the responsibilities and the possible errors that may occur.

Allow me to explain further with an example. At the beginning of my practice as a dermatologist and enrolled therefore at the Colegio Médico del Distrito Federal, one fine day I received a "united work case"* at my private consulting room. The case was an infant who had developed keloids having suffered extensive burns from boiling oil to a large percentage of their dermic area. The doctor who had examined the child (he was not a dermatologist but acted as though he were one) made the correct diagnosis, but prescribed the wrong treatment, which was to apply dry ice (carbon dioxide snow) to the keloid, and which one supposes given the extent of the keloids involved hundreds of painful applications. On realising that I was not in agreement with the prescribed treatment (which perhaps may have been suitable for keloids of smaller size), I telephoned the chief dermatologist of the unit and explained to him what had happened. He replied that I couldn't undermine the doctor who had prescribed the treatment and that I should continue with the "united work case" exactly as instructed, in the corresponding order, leaving me with little choice but to request that he

* A "united work case" (*unidad de trabajo*) was (and perhaps still is) a *sui generis* agreement between the Instituto Venezolano de los Seguros Sociales or IVSS (Venezuelan Institute of Social Security) and the Federación Médica Venezolana (Venezuelan Medical Federation). Under this agreement insured medical cases were referred to registered dermatologists in their own private practices, which for lack of necessary equipment or instruments, the IVSS were unable to look after themselves.

delete my name from the list of specialists willing to offer this service. That was my first and last "united work case", at the beginning of my medical practice when I needed the money the most. I share this anecdote with you as it reveals the antagonism that can occur between a routine procedure (the "united work case") and an unavoidable principle, in this case the treatment prescribed by a colleague, which I disagreed with. Such disagreements can be routine in a hospital environment where they are resolved by the hierarchical authority, but in this case it turned into a delicate institutional problem. The colleague who made the diagnosis and prescribed the treatment was on the institution's payroll, whereas the dermatologist who happened to be assigned this "united work case" by the aforementioned employee, did not officially belong to the institution and so there existed no "procedure" to amend the mistaken therapeutic treatment. If I did not respect the instructions, then there was no other solution than to resign from the system. I did so without hesitation, whilst leaving no doubt about the strength of my objections, thinking always of the poor child who would be cruelly subjected to a treatment, which in order to have any degree of effectiveness would need to be regularly administered hundreds of times.

This experience alone made me think about the importance of the medical act as a whole and the responsibilities it involves.

16th Paradox
Clinic vs. Laboratory

Back when I was studying medicine, more than half a century ago now for I received my medico-surgical diploma in 1951, my teachers and better still my masters (masters being those who teach by their own example in addition to the material within their remit), always insisted that whilst laboratory tests were an important accessory, they were always subordinate to the judgement, knowledge and experience of the clinician who interpreted a series of factors before reaching a diagnosis and prescribing a treatment.

Throughout history, medicine has generated controversy, if not genuine conflict, amongst factions with different points of view about its practice. Some of these are familiar to us, for example: bedside clinical science versus laboratory science; practice skills versus research skills; technical pre-qualifications versus humanistic pre-qualifications when assessing the suitability of medical studies; generalists versus specialists; practical doctors versus academics (in the teaching sense); universities versus hospitals versus research institutions.

New medical technology, especially in the field of imagery, permits access to an extraordinary wealth of information and offers great precision in its indications. This means that it represents a real temptation to put careful clinical judgement to one side in favour of being led by the results offered by sophisticated machines; machines which modern technology is producing in an inexhaustible cornucopia.

In 1981 an editorial in *The Lancet* stated: "The comforting, if spurious, precision of laboratory results have the same attraction as a life jacket to the poor swimmer", going on to explain the reasons for which doctors order so many unnecessary tests: there is the "just in case" test requested by the young doctor "just in case" the consultant asks for it, and the "routine test", the results of which rarely contribute to the diagnosis, and the "aha" test, the results of which were known as abnormal in certain illnesses and which were ordered to "promote the skill of the clinician". "This phenomenon of 'over-investigation', the undertaking of a large number of tests on patients whose medical problems are very apparent, may appear to be a rather trivial matter, but it is costly, and more seriously, it introduces a bizarre element to the medical encounter, by degrading the importance of wisdom and experience in favour of a spurious objectivity."

In the context of malpractice lawsuits and a desire to "watch one's back", unnecessary tests are ordered. For example, in dermatology the clinical diagnosis of basal cell carcinoma is a matter of routine, which makes a preliminary biopsy and histopathological tests unnecessary in the definitive treatment of the illness. However, in consideration of the legal risks and in order to avoid complaints of such a disagreeable nature, it is frequently advisable to obtain a test in case of the need for a more "radical" treatment than usual.

17th Paradox
Essential examinations vs. Optional examinations

There are instrumental examinations and laboratory tests that are indispensable to the establishment of a certain diagnosis, and based on said diagnosis, the ability to lay the foundations of an adequate treatment.

However, it is easy to exaggerate that necessity and order a plethora of explorations and examinations that won't contribute to changing the diagnosis, thereby needlessly increasing the cost of the medical act.

Some colleagues, perhaps rationalising their behaviour with the thought that many of their patients are insured and will therefore not directly cover this increase in costs themselves, have no qualms whatsoever in ordering redundant examinations in order to try to confirm or reinforce their suspected diagnoses. Other colleagues justify it by thinking it prudent to order tests as a precaution and as proof of their professional competency against possible medical malpractice lawsuits. In the long run, it is a negative factor that contributes to the increase of costs to unsustainable levels.

This overuse can reach extremes that are hard to justify. I recall the case of a patient who, after a fall, had a suspected shoulder fracture. The consulted orthopaedic surgeon ordered a magnetic resonance scan of the area and, without a prior examination, also suggested immediate surgical intervention. Fortunately, a second opinion revealed, first clinically and then with the support of an X-ray test, that the fracture could be treated successfully with appropriate immobilisation.

18th Paradox
Satisfaction vs. Dissatisfaction in medical practice

Medical studies are capable of attracting the best young students of a generation: the most intelligent, the most capable, the hardest working, the most ambitious, and the most upstanding people of both sexes. And yet the future security of our profession depends in great part on the level of satisfaction and "fulfilment" felt by its active professionals, their chosen career must in some way be a balance between their expectations and its reality.

Although there are still no serious irreversible signs, a certain reduction in admission levels reveals a degree of dissatisfaction in current trends. The interpretation that I consider to be closest to reality is that what the new generation of doctors resent most, more than the meagre economic compensation disproportionate to the level of effort, concentration and time that the job demands of the doctor, is the "loss of control" itself, subordinate as doctors are to the rules established by the insurers and/or the hospital administration. It is a situation that must be resolved sooner rather than later, as it may eventually cause the medical profession to lose the favour that it once enjoyed from those tempted to pursue it as a life's career. It is also important to remember that it is not, in essence, a lucrative way to make a living, nor is it a priesthood, and if the society which it serves wishes to continue having access to good doctors, it will have to realise that doctors must regain at least some of the control that they once had over medical decisions concerning their patients.

If this trend is not corrected, medicine as a profession will gradually, but inexorably, miss out on the most talented young people of every new generation. This is something that, until only a short time ago, we took for granted, for medicine was always slated by numerous surveys in the most advanced countries as the first choice career of the most gifted secondary school students. If we are not capable of attracting the best students, medicine will not manage to achieve the ambitious goals that its leaders and drivers have proposed, objectives that are undoubtedly ambitious but achievable only in so much as we currently have the key element at our disposal: the best human resources available.

This is a problem that certainly did not "kill the dream" of our profession's leadership on a worldwide level in the immediate past, but it should worry those who currently have this responsibility, who should seriously reconsider the corrections required to revert a trend that is presently barely visible, but the consequences of which may be extremely grave for the future of medicine and its traditional role in society.

To complicate the situation further, in parallel and clear competition with doctors of orthodox training, we have the recent graduation in Venezuela of new professionals, with the grandiose title of "*médicos integrales comunitarios*" (MIC) (Primary Community Physicians). These MICs, with their reduced study plan of Cuban design, improvised teachers, an absence of well-established selection and dubious suitability for hospital work, will have a negative influence on future candidates for our profession, who easily sense a depreciated activity, undermined by future work conflicts between two types of professionals with very different academic training. It is feasible to imagine that mistakes in diagnosis and treatment by these MIC doctors, fruits of improvisation in a sector that does not allow it, will discredit the medical profession as a whole in the eyes of the general public. It is clear that faced with such a situation, orthodox medical studies will lose the great attraction that they once held.

19th Paradox
Traditional information vs. Information sourced from the Internet

The patient's level of knowledge about medicine and their illness always influences the communication between doctor and patient. It is natural and logical that the patient will ask the treating doctor for a minimum of information about the illness, its causes, its development, their prognosis, treatment and possible consequences. Until recently, the patient (bar rare exceptions, usually if the patient was a doctor him- or herself or if related to a doctor) would accept the treating doctor's concise explanation without hesitation, or even many questions, with the dialogue being brief and limited to the instructions given by the doctor.

With easy domestic access to websites via a computer and the Internet, these days it is common that, even before seeking a doctor's appointment – especially if a certain diagnosis is already suspected – the patient will be well-documented about the ailment and may have even prepared, at least mentally, a number of pertinent questions which, according to the answers that they receive, may permit the formation of a judgement about their practitioner's current knowledge. In reality, perhaps subconsciously, the patient carries out a sort of "preliminary examination" of the doctor, which is part of a type of initial evaluation to determine if the chosen professional has the expertise they would expect.

This evaluation, based on a single search through rather disorganised online information and interpreted by a person who lacks the basic background information indispensible to a full understanding of the problem, however simply it is attempted to be expressed, can clearly lead to multiple confusions and mistaken judgements on the part of the patient. These days doctors must have this reality in mind, as every new patient may already be informed about their possible illness and wish to assess the current knowledge of their chosen practitioner, via the aforementioned method. This in itself is not a negative characteristic of this new style of medical practice, apart from the fact that a lack of preparation in many people, as already indicated, can lead to a confusion of ideas that the doctor must try to clarify.

Websites offer an unparalleled extraordinary richness of information; currently many searchers (personally Google is my favourite search engine) have the issue of knowing how to navigate the veritable "jungle" of information available in order to break down the superfluous from the fundamental. It is not an easy task. *The Doctor's Guide to the Internet* written by Robert Kiley* and published by the Royal Society of Medicine in London, is very useful for doctors in the complex search for relevant information online.

In contrast with these benefits, we should mention that the lack of any type of control or filter could lead to the spread of erroneous or even badly intentioned information. Hence the importance of supporting the information with a reference to its intellectual authorship, usually along with the academic and/or hospital affiliations of the author, which permits the reader an understanding of the reliability of the information.

* Robert Kiley, British librarian, Head of Digital Services at the Wellcome Library in London

20th Paradox
Insurance institutions vs. The medical profession

The so-called "health industry" has come to be by far the largest economic industry in the world's biggest power, the United States of America. In spite of its enormous health expenditure, the North American system is far from being the most efficient, not least in its ability to cover the minimum medical requirements of the whole population, and there is deep social dissatisfaction at the lack of ability to fully carry out a task that is considered a right by modern society. At the beginning of the new millennium it was estimated that there were 41 million Americans without health insurance cover (the cost of which is in the vicinity of 88 billion dollars a year). As the population of the United States at that time was 270 million, this means that 15% of its population was lacking any kind of insurance to afford them adequate medical attention. The great paradox lies in the fact that this is happening in a country that spends more on health than anywhere else in the world.

The problem is not just limited to the evident necessity for the whole population to have some sort of medical insurance, but also that in highly "litigant" societies such as the United States, no doctor can practise their profession without malpractice insurance to protect them against claims attempted rationally and justifiably, or by patients who are dissatisfied with or harmed by the medical act. The increase in premiums of this type of insurance for doctors is responsible for the increase in their fees. This phenomenon is particularly noticeable in the states of California, New York and Florida. In this first state, in 1985 the services of an obstetrician were in the order of 82,500 dollars and 101,000 dollars for a neurosurgeon.

As with new technology, this is a factor in continual increase. One of the negative consequences of this situation is that doctors prefer to abandon treatments with low rates of success. This leads to an excessively prudent medical practice, which can be dramatically harmful to those who suffer from certain illnesses.

It is important to emphasise that in many cases it is the insurers who determine which treatment is pursued for many people.

It is still a little premature to judge if the recent Obama-led reforms of the North American health system, or Obamacare as they are known, which were intended to eliminate or at least considerably diminish the number of patients without medical insurance, will have the expected beneficial effects.

21st Paradox
The pharmaceutical industry vs. The medical profession

Until very recently, in spite of the accumulated knowledge of the natural history of illnesses and their signs and symptoms, the therapeutic arsenal of doctors was restricted to bloodletting, gastric juices and purgatives without any scientific proof of their effectiveness. In the nineteenth century, advances in clinical examinations with a good clinical history, pathological anatomy and microbiology became the fundamentals for an accurate diagnosis. However, beyond a few inoculations, Salvarsan for syphilis, quinine for malaria, digitalis for heart weakness and various sedatives and painkillers (principally aspirin), doctors had very little to offer their patients.

With the birth and exponential growth of the pharmaceutical industry, from the end of the nineteenth century to the present day, its economic power has had a two-way influence on doctors. On the one hand, it decidedly contributes to providing us with therapeutic weapons, which are increasingly effective, sophisticated and specific. On the other hand, in order to determine the efficiency of their patented pharmaceuticals and above all to effectively trade their products, pharmaceutical companies have no hesitation in attempting to obtain the collaboration of physicians for their clinical tests. They therefore seek preference for their pharmaceuticals, through timeworn procedures, such as dispensing discretionary favours (like covering the expenses of attending conferences and other meetings of a scientific nature), which can occasionally result in problems of an ethical nature.

The subject of the pharmaceutical industry offering doctors "favours" has been widely discussed in the main medical journals. As a significant example let us refer to the *British Medical Journal* editorial from 31 May 2003, entitled: "No more free lunches", which categorises some of the many favours received. The editors of the magazine state: "Doctors and drug companies must work together, but doctors do not need to be banqueted, transported in luxury, put up in the best hotels, and educated by drug companies. The result is bias in the decisions made about patient care. Drug companies are commercial companies that must market their products. Sometimes they bend the rules, but it is doctors who are perhaps more to blame in coming to depend on drug company largesse. How did we reach the point where doctors expect their information, research, education, professional organisations, and attendance at conferences to be underwritten by drug companies? Both doctors and drug companies know there is something unhealthy in this relationship, but seem unable to stop themselves."

It ends by saying: "The pharmaceutical industry is immensely powerful. It is one of the most profitable of industries, truly global, and closely connected to politicians, particularly in the United States. Compared with it, medicine is a disorganised mess. Doctors have become dependent on the industry in a way that undermines their independence and ability to do their best by patients. Medical reform groups in the United States are calling for this greater distance in relationships with industry and for independent education and sources of information. The University of California is considering ending free lunches sponsored by drug companies, and American medical students are being asked to take a revised Hippocratic oath that forbids the accepting of money, gifts, or hospitality. These are moves that doctors worldwide should follow." (Abbasi & Smith, 2003: 1155–6)

As an example of the economic importance of the pharmaceutical industry, let's take the case of the United States, the largest economy in the world, with a pharmaceutical industry that made profits in the order of 99.5 billion dollars in 1998, an increase of 11% from the year before. Global sales also increased 7% in the year 1997/98 alone, making the pharmaceutical industry the fastest growing, with the largest legitimate profits in the whole world.

In 1953, in the United States alone there were 140,000 medicinal products listed for sale, 75% of them introduced in the previous ten years. Between 1929 and 1969, prescription drugs expenditure increased by 25%, from 190 million dollars to 5.3 billion dollars.§ Nothing gives a better idea of the public "intoxication" (medical profession included) with the new and powerful medicines than the fact that in 1945, the year in which penicillin was made truly accessible to the greater public, it was administered to one in four North Americans. It will certainly have saved many lives, but it is likely that it has been used unnecessarily in thousands of cases.

The research and development of new pharmaceuticals relies on the high purchasing power markets of the industrialised nations of the developed world. In 1998, the United States alone had a budget that amounted to 17 billion dollars. It is important to note that "pharmaceutical firms operate like any private industry and they don't have any specific social mission, responding to economic imperatives more than those of a social or humanitarian nature."

It is estimated that the average cost of the research and development involved in putting a new drug on the market is in the region of 500 million dollars, and that the company that makes this investment aspires to recuperate their costs over a period of three to five years through the sale of the product, with the aim of generating profits by the closing of this period.

§ *Alfred Kopf, MD: It is worth mentioning the very high cost of some of the new biologics (i.e., isolated from a variety of natural sources such as human; animal; microorganisms rather than chemically synthesized). For example, the cost of one year of induction and maintenance for some of the biologics for the treatment of psoriasis is over $50,000. Who can afford this?*

With these figures, it's easy to conclude that only the largest multi-nationals of the United States, Switzerland, Germany, Great Britain, France and Japan, can successfully compete in this industry, which, with no interest in the tropical illnesses of poor countries, attends only to the market needs of affluent countries. We have to mention that this imbalance is at least partially, and quite rightly, redressed by programmes of the World Health Organisation (WHO) and donations of various large international foundations, especially by the Wellcome Trust in Great Britain, which has always had the good judgement to dedicate a significant part of its funds to tropical medicine research.

To explain the insatiable "appetite" of human beings for medicine we must remember the aphorism of Sir William Osler when he declared: "The desire to take medicine is perhaps the greatest feature which distinguishes man from animals." (Osler, cited in Cushing, 1940: 342)

22nd Paradox
Politicians vs. The medical profession

Given that health is the issue that most concerns the population, it is little wonder that politicians promise the earth in health matters during electoral campaigns in order to gain the public vote. This can negatively affect doctors' work, and working relationships between the medical profession and governments are increasingly difficult and complex, requiring the almost daily intervention of the medical profession, grouped as it is into colleges and federations.

A notable case is the "the right to health" (instead of "the right to medical aid"), which is included in the "Bolivarian" Republic of Venezuela's new Constitution, where the State "guarantees" the health of all Venezuelans. Is this ignorance, naivety, cynicism or demagogy, or perhaps a combination of all four?

The close relationship between politics and medicine is immediately clear when one becomes aware of the intimate and inextricable relationship between, on the one hand, the health and well-being of citizens and, on the other hand, a government's political decisions. The German pathologist Rudolf Virchow (1821–1902) stands out amongst those who most keenly understood this. He went so far as to think of politics as one of medicine's many branches, in so much as it has a duty to ensure certain aspects of human well-being, whilst medicine encompasses all aspects.

Virchow applied the cellular theory of pathology and proclaimed the new doctrine of *omnis cellula e cellula* (every cell originates in another cell). A key figure in German politics of his time, as a man of liberal vision he opposed the great statistician and chancellor of Prussia (and from 1870 the new German Empire) Prince Otto von Bismarck

(1815–98). His many, often funny, anecdotes are still well-known today. Here is one of them:

Bismarck, supposedly troubled by Virchow's criticism, challenged him to a duel. As the challenged party, Virchow had the right to choose the weapons and arrived at the field of honour with a beautiful case. The patrons and witnesses were horrified that Virchow had selected pistols to settle the conflict, for they were all aware of Bismarck's reputation for weapon handling and his experience as a dueller (at least a sword would give Virchow some chance of survival after the first blood had been spilled). To the surprise of everyone present, what was actually enclosed in the case was a pair of sausages, identical in appearance. To the astonishment of all present, Virchow explained that one was a deadly weapon as it had been contaminated with lethal bacteria chosen by Virchow himself, the other was perfectly innocuous. "Let's allow his Excellency to decide which one he wishes to eat, and I will eat the other", said Virchow. Needless to say the "Iron Chancellor" withdrew from the duel.

As well as a way of making fun of duels as a conflict resolution method, Virchow used it as an opportunity to demonstrate once and for all that the person who sets a goal, of this type or of any other nature, thinks that they have the advantage (which nearly always turns out to be true), which explains their supposed courage and bravery.

On my request, Luis Enrique Alcalá* has contributed the following:

"I'm grateful to you for bringing the new edition of *Medical Paradoxes* to my attention. Below I enclose some lines that you may edit liberally according to how they suit your publication.

* Luis Enrique Alcalá, Venezuelan sociologist and political analyst

"In various articles from my blog I recognise the fact that I owe any information on the political-medical approach of Virchow to you. For example, in *Enfermo de pobreza* (Sick of Poverty), I said:

"It was the illustrious dermatologist and ex-Ambassador Francisco Kerdel-Vegas, tireless builder of Venezuelanness,* who alerted me to the political views of Rudolf Virchow, the great German pathologist who equally served as a parliamentarian in his country. He viewed politics as an activity of a medical nature. The context of this invaluable information was a conversation in which I explained to Dr Kerdel that this had been my express perspective since 1984. (Alcalá, 2006)

"During that meeting at my house (in November 1984 with Diego Bautista Urbaneja and Gerardo Cabañas), I explained for the first time my sense of the road ahead for our legitimisation as politicians on a "medical" road. I called it "the medical metaphor". The political act is a medical act, I said, as it is fundamentally about proposing, selecting and applying treatments to problems. (Alcalá, 2008)

"At the beginning of the following year, 1985, I received a copy of one of Yehezkel Dror's works . . . In one of them Dror, a friend and teacher since 1972, said the following: '. . . policy sciences are, in part, a clinical profession and craft.' (. . .) His position was only slightly less radical than mine, given that what interested me was the conceptual territory that is exactly defined by that part that is a profession and a 'clinical' art (. . .). (Alcalá, 1986)

"The image or metaphor of political medicine is not entirely original to me. I received Yehezkel Dror's aforementioned work some months after the statement I made to my previously mentioned friends, as it is also true that the focus of my proposition is displaced by the partial

* Translator's note: the word Venezuelanness is the translation of the invented word *Venezolanidad*, which is intended to give the sense of somebody who is proud of and wishes to promote the Venezuelan national character

admission of Yehezkel. However, something from the reading of one of his books, *Design for Policy Sciences*, must have remained in my unconscious memory. From 1971, it says: '. . . the analogue between policy sciences and medicine is nevertheless a very suggestive one, because of strong similarities in some of the main paradigms and secondary characteristics'. On the same point I cite René Dubois, who in *Man, Medicine and Environment* says the following: '. . . Medicine seems best suited to preside in an architectonic way over the development of a new science of human life.' (Alcalá, 1986)

"(At the end of 2002, I began work on a weekly letter on political issues, using from that point forward the 'brand' Dr Político in order to indicate that I understand Politics as an art of medical character. Ten years later, Radio Caracas gave me a weekly slot that transmits under the name Dr Político. It was during a friendly lunch in mid-2004 that Dr Francisco Kerdel-Vegas told me that Rudolf Virchow, the great German pathologist, believed he was practising medicine when working as a member of the Reichstag in regions of his country. In 2005, Jeffrey Sachs published his book *The End of Poverty*, the fourth chapter of which was entitled 'Clinical Economics'; in 1993, the Venezuelan economist José Toro Hardy organised his *Fundamentos de Teoría Económica* (Foundations of Economic Theory) as a medical treatise. 'In an attempt to facilitate comprehension of economics, it seemed fitting to suggest that this be focused in the same way as medicine is studied.' But it was none other than Jorge Luis Borges who said: 'One creates one's own precursors.' What is clear is that the medicalparadigm of Politics is out there, and that is because it works.)"

23rd Paradox
Rational use vs. Abusive and convenient use of intensive care units

Intensive care units have been a built-in part of all general hospitals for a number of decades. Back in 1852 Florence Nightingale (1820–1920), in her significant visionary role as founder of nursing as an important component of joint health professional services, declared that it was of particular value "to have one place in the hospital where post-operative and other patients needing close attention can be watched." (Jennett, 1985)

Intensive care units are precisely where everything that cutting-edge technology represents is most obviously displayed to the public, with their modern monitoring and resuscitation equipment, computers etc., giving the impression that the adequate and opportune use of this group of diverse and complex apparatus can signify the difference between life and death. In spite of the fact that numerous statistical studies tend to demonstrate to the contrary, I have no doubt that the balance must be favourable for whilst in the beginning the units were perhaps a new "fashion", one of the many that periodically invade medicine, they have become institutionalised and constitute an important part of a modern hospital.

Perhaps the issue lies more in the appropriate use of the unit than in the questioning of its existence for correctly monitoring those patients who require close and careful observation, either because they have had a heart attack or because they are in the immediate postoperative period.§

§ *Alfred Kopf, MD: Intensive Care Units are for inpatients who have developed serious medical problems. Another problem hospitals face is the escalating costs for a patient to attend outpatient "Emergency Rooms" in hospitals. Today, many*

Given the level of sophistication of the equipment in use and the need for the constant human presence of doctors and paramedical personnel to monitor it, the cost for the hospital is very high and this translates into highly elevated fees for the patient staying there. There is a clear divorce between what can be beneficial, and even vital, for the gravely ill patient, and what is financially affordable for the patient or their family (given the gravity of the cases admitted, it is likely that many will die there). In an anecdotal capacity I recall a colleague who wore a medal of sorts hung from his collar – similar to those used by soldiers for identification during the last world war – with the engraved instructions: "Under no circumstances must I be admitted to an intensive care unit," perhaps thinking that although his life may be saved, the unpleasant experience would signify the partial or total loss of his life savings, and if he were to die, the disagreeable prospect of leaving his family to inherit a considerable debt.

I also recall the description of a unit of this type in the highly critical writing of Dr Vernon Coleman in his previously quoted book:
". . . the patient who goes into a coronary-care unit will be treated like a battery hen. He will be tied up to a row of frightening machines and deprived of all contact with the real world. Instead of comfort, sympathy and understanding, he will be surrounded by cold, clinical, computerized efficiency. The intensive care unit is designed for doctors, not patients. It is a perfect breeding ground for research papers. It is a terrible place for a sick patient." (Coleman, 1989: 84–5)

(continued from previous page)
patients go to outpatient Emergency Rooms for a number of problems, some simple, some emergent. They utilize these facilities because of the ease of access and inability to see their private doctors for one reason or another. Many hospitals will accept any patient, even those who cannot afford to pay. Thus, the hospitals have to absorb such deficits or find funds elsewhere to cover these costs, which currently have skyrocketed; just another increasing problem for our hospitals.

By 1995 the cost of intensive care units in the United States had escalated to the impressive amount of 62 billion dollars (equivalent to 1% of the GDP of the country), a third of which (20 billion) was spent on what came to be euphemistically called PIC (potentially ineffective care).

There is an important element to consider: the convenience of the doctor. Expending valuable time in a car, traversing a complicated journey with confusing directions and visiting different addresses is not the same as concentrating all patients in a critical state in the same place where they are accustomed to working and, moreover, have at their disposal a delegate of efficient supervision that can be controlled with timely phone calls.

Recent studies reveal the bitter reality that the medical cost of the last days of a patient's life is higher than that of the cost of the whole of his or her life up to that point.

24th Paradox
Increase in number of doctors vs. Growth of dissatisfaction with their services

With the continual growth of specialisms and sub-specialisms in medicine, there is a tendency for patients to be referred in order to seek additional useful information to corroborate a diagnosis and establish a treatment. This translates into more appointments and waiting, additional fees and very often the need to visit other surgeries, even other clinics and hospitals. It is what is known in the playful slang of the Venezuelan vernacular as *peloteo* (a rally or a football being kicked back and forth). It all leads to trouble and annoyance for the patients who view it as "passing the ball from one doctor to another", a procedure that is often unjustified and costly. The moral of this is the same as it always is: the interests of the patient must be kept in mind and the inconvenience of such referrals should be as limited as possible.

It is often the case that dissatisfaction is not directly related to the medical attention itself, but rather to the organisation of the whole process – for example, long waits at the surgery, or waiting to be admitted or registered at a clinic – a situation that doesn't just affect free public services but has extended into private medicine too.

These referrals can also be interpreted as evading and diluting the responsibility of the diagnosis and "recovery through health", that is to say preventatively. Faced with the potential of malpractice appeals from patients, doctors cover themselves by seeking the coinciding opinion of another physician.

Doctors are also dissatisfied with the omnipresent incursions by those diverse sectors of society trying to regulate the medical act, whether politicians, hospital administrations, insurance company actuaries or simply patients who have self-diagnosed online, undoubtedly with indigestion from an excess of information that has not been "digested" by a mind prepared by many years of dedicated and methodical study. Dealing with such a great number of opinions based on casual information, and frequently without scientific basis, requires holy patience.

The establishment of a dichotomy in the medical profession is foreseeable for the future in those countries like Venezuela that have tried with little success, if any, to train doctors via accelerated programmes without the necessary hospital experience and with teachers whose training could only be described as improvised. In Venezuela this has resulted in the so-called Primary Community Physicians or MICs* (based on Cuban experience); these doctors will compete in the market with doctors who have had traditional training via selective universities, demanding programmes and well-trained teachers. And so there is the establishment of an inevitable dichotomy in the medical profession, from every undesirable, and even dangerous, point of view.

It is clear that the governmental authorities responsible for such medical education public policy dismiss, at their temporary convenience, the 1,000-year-old experience represented by medical training. It is fairly obvious that this is a highly delicate, sensitive and risky matter for, as with every educational experiment, the possibly negative results will take a long time to demonstrate their value or inefficiency as they can only be established and tested over a prolonged period of several years. A change of this type, when it's about health and even people's lives, represents a high-risk somersault. This can all result in great confusion for the public, above all in the public sector where people have been inundated by official propaganda to such an extent that they have come to believe that Primary Community Physicians are sufficiently trained and experienced enough to trust them with their lives.

* See Paradox 18 for an explanation of these

25th Paradox
Inferiority complex vs. Objective evaluation of our reality and our potential

This is in fact a universal problem that covers all imaginable situations and manifests itself in the most subtle and versatile behaviour; due to its ubiquity this includes medicine too. For our generation it occurs predominately in everything related to medicine from the United States. Given the undeniably advanced technological progress of this country, it is not uncommon to come across criticism, with undeniable foundation, of what appear to be clear failures and defects in the North American public health coverage system. What is regrettable is when the extremes of absurd and counterproductive paranoia are reached, and a puerile inventiveness is used to justify and endorse actions and positions that border on the ridiculous. Allow me to explain with a striking example. I recall a letter received from a distinguished North American lecturer and researcher, it must have been towards the end of 1979 or at the beginning of 1980. The letter gave me a brief explanation of the discovery in San Francisco of a new variety of Kaposi's haemorrhagic sarcoma (histopathologically demonstrated) in young and promiscuous homosexuals, and put forward the hypothesis that it could be a new contagious disease, possibly produced by a virus. The purpose of this communication, as well as alerting me to the problem, was to find out if we had observed anything similar in Venezuela. I immediately replied that I had not come across any similar cases, but taking into account the importance of the communication and its author, I made three copies of the letter and sent them to the Minister of Health and Social Welfare, the President of the National Academy of Medicine and the President of the Venezuelan Dermatology Society. As expected, I didn't receive a single reply. However, just a few days later one of the most highly circulated newspapers in Caracas published a report on an epidemiologist press conference where it was more or less stated that information relating to a supposed new disease "invented" by the North Americans had come to light (probably one of the copies of the letter that I circulated). This almost certainly had the intention of distracting the attention of underdeveloped countries from their real public health problems. As it is easy to conclude, my North American colleague had informed me of the beginning of the great pandemic of the century: AIDS. It was not an imperialist "invention" intended to damage us. Fortunately, at least in this particular case, there was no evident damage caused to the population by this biased view of reality, but it did leave me very concerned because it proved once again the eternal complex that reaches the extremes of imagining conspiracies in the field of collective health.

26th Paradox
Humility vs. Arrogance and dogma

Although this is a general human behaviour problem, it has special meaning in the case of doctors. We must learn from the many errors committed in the past and assume a less dogmatic and arrogant attitude when faced with new ideas and concepts. Whilst nobody is burned at the stake for supporting ideas outside of the current dogma anymore, it is possible that medicine's progress is delayed by rigid attitudes founded in established ideas when faced with new evidence to the contrary.

To understand the levels to which this attitude can go, one only has to remember the French National Academy of Medicine's unfavourable opinion of the discovery of anaesthesia in Boston.

Most new ideas have initially been fought, often in a highly treacherous way. The reactions of "the establishment" when faced with the discoveries of Harvey, Galvani, Semmelweis, Claude Bernard, Pasteur, Golgi, Freud, etc. are well-known by all, as discussed in depth by the North American journalist and writer Hal Hellman.

A vivid telling of the difficulties of putting forward a new concept that contradicts the pre-established dogma is found in the pages of *Dr Folkman's War* by Robert Cooke.

These struggles often end in tragedy, as was certainly the case with my colleague and dear and admired friend Dr René Favaloro.

It is well-known that Argentine citizen Doctor Favaloro both disseminated and proved the value of the coronary bypass when he was working at the Cleveland Clinic in the United States; an operation that benefits hundreds of thousands of people with heart disease every year. His work, inventiveness, knowledge and creativity were recognised throughout the world, (chairs of cardiovascular surgery were baptised in his name in Moscow and Tel Aviv). René Favaloro could have stayed in the United States where he would likely have received many generous and attractive offers of work. However, his social sensibility and patriotism impeded him from doing so and he felt he should return to Buenos Aires to offer the benefit of his experience to his compatriots. As a means of disseminating and adequately using his knowledge and experience, he established a whole system there: a foundation, hospital and university. He got himself into debt to do it and when he realised that those people and institutions (especially his country's government) that had promised to collaborate with him to help the poor were not going to fulfil their promise, he simply took his own life. The painful consequence of a soul that was deeply sensitive to the grave problems of the poor. Perhaps this is a lesson to be learned by our frivolous and consumerist society.*

The stereotype of the kind-hearted, generous, humble doctor who is only interested in the well-being of their patients (well-established by the Venezuelans and their Antille neighbours between them in the figure of Dr José Gregorio Hernández (1864–1919)), is contrasted with that of the arrogant, materialistic and worldly doctor who is the object of endless jokes by satirical and biting critics such as Jean-Baptiste Molière (1622–73) and George Bernard Shaw (1856–1950).

As medicine has become more scientific, doctors have shown a tendency to be more arrogant, interpreting the advances of science applied to human health as an exceptional power – which it is – with which all problems can be resolved, including the greatest unknown

* Dr Rubén Jaén Centeno's interesting book *Aunque la naturaleza se opuso* (Although Nature Objected) clearly explains that the surgical intervention of the coronary bypass was in fact invented in 1962 by the Russian surgeon Vladmir Kolesof in Leningrad (now St Petersburg). So Favaloro was not the inventor of the procedure, but instead made it known worldwide.

of all: which has been hidden from us until now in the functioning of the human brain.

Only when science achieves separation from the metaphysical and magical does it come to represent a driving force for modern civilisation. However, even in this era of great promise in scientific advancement we must keep in mind the words of perhaps the most important scientist of all time, for science obtained its current indisputable credibility and supremacy through his contributions, Sir Isaac Newton (1642–1727): "I do not know what I may seem to the world, but to myself, I seem to have been only like a boy playing on the seashore, and diverting myself in now and then finding a smoother pebble or a prettier shell than ordinary, whilst the great ocean of truth lay all undiscovered before me." (Newton cited in Mandelbrote, 2001: 9)

27th Paradox
The right to life vs. The right to abortion

This is a markedly thorny topic as it goes close to the heart of the teachings and dogma of religious principles, especially Catholic ones.

If an unborn child is still human, that is to say a person, the principles of justice, if correctly interpreted, and of not doing harm, prohibit abortion or any procedure or technique carried out with the intention of killing or ending the development of a child who has not yet been born.

From a medical point of view the most agonising problem is when it is believed that an abortion can save the mother's life, a situation that brings to the fore the issue of the mother's right to life vs. the right to life of a creature that has not yet been born. So-called "therapeutic abortion" is justified by the current legislation of numerous countries.

It is interesting to note how Marxism uninhibitedly handled problems that concerned ethical values. Take the Soviet Union where abortion was legal from 1920 to 1936, was declared illegal from 1936 to 1955 and was then legal again in 1955. All of these changes were made in accordance with demographic policies decided on by the government and to meet the perceived needs of the State; in the era of "illegality" repopulation was necessary in order to meet the challenges of industrialisation and to recuperate from the enormous loss of human lives during war.

28th Paradox
Social security vs. Private medicine

In 1881 the Chancellor of the German Empire Otto von Bismarck (1815–98) introduced his legislation on social security in Germany, supposedly as a reaction to the political agitation of socialists in that country, and the just claim by the working class about the risks of disease, medical attention, hospitalisation, death, etc. Ever since this date, there has not been any country in the world that has not attempted a social security scheme of sorts, whether successful or not. It is undoubtedly a social advance of great importance for the working population of a country, but when its administration is monopolised by the State the system gives way to innumerable abuses of all types, that indirectly involve the medical profession, given that an important part of the scheme is based on medical services.

The unscrupulous and, frankly, at times corrupt politicians' management of funds that are based on workers' savings has been a real disgrace in many countries, such as Venezuela. This has contributed to the discrediting of social security, which is one of the most necessary institutions in current society.

I have closely observed the working of the National Health Service of Great Britain for many years and I must express my admiration for everything that it represents. Although it's natural and human that its users point out its defects and above all the delays that it undoubtedly suffers, in general it is a system that works, one that even the Conservative UK government of Margaret Thatcher (1925–2013) decided not to privatise and break up, and rightly so considering that it represents a valuable asset and a social conquest of our era. It should be remembered that a private medicine system for those with the economic means, and who wish to pay, functions in parallel.

My dear friend and classmate (Class of Pastor Orpeza at

Universidad Central de Venezuela, 1951) Antonio Clemente, who has dedicated a large part of his professional life to the subject of social security, sent me the following commentary:

"Social Security is understood as the combination of forward-thinking measures that lead to guaranteeing the inhabitants of a country the economic means to achieve the minimum conditions of comfort, health, education and recreation necessary to civilised man; and the steps against a series of inherent risks in modern life such as unemployment, work-related illness or illness of another origin, partial or complete disability, old age, the education of children and the consequences of the death of the head of a family.

"The first person in history to use the concept in this particular sense was the Liberator Simón Bolívar at the Angostura Congress (15 February 1819), when he said: 'The most perfect governmental system is that which produces the greatest happiness possible, the greatest social security and the greatest political stability.'

"The International Social Security Association (ISSA) is based at the headquarters of the International Labour Organisation (ILO) in Geneva. Until 2002 they published their findings for all countries in one book, from 2002 they split them into four books: 1: Europe, 2: Asia, 3: Africa, and 4: The Americas, this last one has 36 countries or territories.

"The information is processed by the International Social Security Association (ISSA), which has been going for 75 years. It is checked and edited by the Social Security Administration of the United States (SSA).§ The first edition was published in 1937. The system is based on the contribution of: 1: Businesses (65%), 2: Workers (25%) and 3: The State (10%). These are averages and vary between countries."

§ *Alfred Kopf, MD: In the USA there is a differentiation between the financial aspects (Social Security) and the medical aspects (Medicare, Medicaid, Obama care, and a number of other specific medical coverages for the nation). How this relates to the global governmental services must be puzzling.*

29th Paradox
Today's truth vs. Tomorrow's lies

This has already been expressed in a highly lucid way by Sir William Osler with the words: "The philosophies of one age have become the absurdities of the next, and the foolishness of yesterday has become the wisdom of tomorrow; through long ages which we're slowly learning what we are hurrying to forget – amid all the changes and chances of twenty-five centuries, the profession has never lacked men who have lived up to these Greeks ideals." (Osler, 1902)

The way in which the pendulum swings in everything related to what could be called "the prevalent wisdom of the moment", changing as frequently as women's fashion, is common knowledge.

After all, these days who remembers bloodletting, purging, induced vomiting, colon cleansing, artificial pneumothorax, or scarification and cupping (these last two were still in use in my generation)?

30th Paradox
Clinical medicine vs. Molecular medicine

There is good reason to hope that within a relatively short period of time we will be able to positively act on many of the diseases caused by the particular genetic anomalies that can be identified at a molecular level. Such is the case with sickle-cell anaemia, caused by a single "error" in the deoxyribonucleic acid (DNA), or cystic fibrosis.

Molecular medicine (molecular biology department) is nothing but pure and simple medicine. It is a new frontier focused on the treatment and cure of diseases, as well as disease prevention and the general promotion of health.

The progress achieved in this direction in the last few years is truly extraordinary. The discovery in Cambridge of the double helix shape of the DNA molecule in 1953 by Francis Crick* and James D. Watson[†] signalled the beginning of a new era.

15 April 2003 was auspiciously announced by international news agencies in celebration of half a century since news of the discovery of the DNA molecular structure was first published in the British journal *Nature*, on 25 April 1953. In the year 2000, two years earlier than anticipated, 99.9% of the human genetic map had been de-codified by a public consortium comprised of scientists from six countries. The project began in 1990 with an initial budget of three billion dollars, to be used over 15 years, however, the experts only used 2.7 billion and by the year 2000 a draft of the code had already been achieved. After three billion years of evolution, we now have before us the series of instructions that every single one of us carries, from the (fertilised) ovary through to adult age and the grave. This is the "book of life", or

* Francis Crick (1916–2004), British molecular biologist
[†] James D. Watson (1928–), American molecular biologist

a genetic map, upon which contemporary science has placed so many hopes, confident of discovering treatments for diseases that were until now incurable or hereditary, treating defective genes, or prescribing specific medicines according to the genetic code of each person. There are 30,000 genes hidden in the tangle of DNA (a single gene can produce up to 98,000 proteins) and 3 billion base pairs, entwined in the long spiral formed by chromosomes.

There are those who doubt the great expectation that has been attributed to the practical applications of this genetic knowledge.

Let's look at the negative view of "the New Genetics" by qualified observer Dr James Le Fanu:

"The New Genetics, in the three distinctive but overlapping applications of genetic engineering, genetic screening and genetic therapy, generates genuinely novel and brilliant answers to fundamental problems. And yet for all the enthusiasm and excitement and the millions of hours of research endeavour and the tens of thousands of scientific papers and the acres of newspaper coverage, its practical benefits are scarcely detectable. Genetic engineering has turned out to be an expensive method of making drugs that were either – like insulin – already available, or have been shown to be of marginal thera-peutic benefit. Genetic screening has had hardly any impact on the prevention of the common inherited disorders, and gene therapy simply does not work. Nor, indeed, is this all, for several other much anticipated benefits of the New Genetics have similarly failed to fulfil the expecta-tions held out for them, most notably the genetic transformation of pigs as a source of organs for transplantation." (Le Fanu, 2011: 345)

31st Paradox
The triumphs vs. The failures of contemporary medicine

From the point of view of preventative medicine, there is no greater triumph than that of the elimination of smallpox. This occurred over the duration of 182 years, which was the period between the discovery of the vaccine and the eradication of the disease. Edward Jenner* presented his original report to the Royal Society in 1797 but it was rejected by the then president Sir Joseph Banks (1743–1820), who was also his personal friend, under the premise that Jenner's ideas were too revolutionary and his experimental evidence too limited. Banks advised Jenner that he shouldn't risk his reputation by presenting findings that appeared to contradict established knowledge at the august institution.

Fortunately, Jenner was not a man to be deterred by the first obstacle in his way and in 1798 he published at his own expense a 64-page pamphlet that described his findings and discovery. On the 8 May 1980, the Assembly of the World Health Organisation met in Geneva and officially declared the definitive eradication of smallpox, thanks to the rational use of the vaccine invented by Jenner nearly two centuries before. I had the opportunity to observe many of the last cases of this dreaded disease in Addis Ababa, the capital of Ethiopia, where I travelled in 1973 in the company of Professors Harvey Blank (of Miami) and Coleman Jacobson (of Dallas). This terrible disease had wreaked havoc on my family. My paternal grandmother had smallpox and her newborn daughter died from it. It is difficult to calculate precisely how many millions of human beings were killed by the smallpox virus, how many were left blind, how many with deforming scars on their face, and, a lesser-known aspect, how it influenced the course of history. What is perfectly well documented is that successive and devastating

* Edward Jenner (1749–1823), British family doctor and poet

epidemics of smallpox in Amerindians, who had previously had no contact with the disease and were therefore virgins immunologically-speaking, contributed to Hernán Cortés' (1485–1547) subjugation of the Aztec Empire between 1519 and 1521, and later assisted Francisco Pizarro (1478–1541) in conquering the Inca Empire (1532). It is estimated that the indigenous population of the Americas, which amounted to 72 million people in 1492 when Christopher Columbus (1451–1506) first stepped ashore, had been decimated by war and diseases (the main one being smallpox) to a total of 600,000 by 1800.

Bizarrely, the potential calamity of smallpox, the only contagious disease to have been eradicated through human action, is far from being completely eliminated as there still exists the danger that it may be used as a weapon of bioterrorism (via cultures grown in a laboratory); for this reason its importance remains current.

The triumphs of medicine in the second half of the twentieth century are extraordinary, above all in everything related to the therapeutic, with the control of diseases that decimated the populations of previous generations, such as tuberculosis and syphilis (at this time leprosy was already being progressively and spontaneously eradicated in Northern countries). However, this bucolic panorama of a promising future was interrupted at the beginning of the 1980s by the AIDS pandemic.

Anybody under the impression that infectious pathogenic diseases are a group of entities that are well-known, limited in number, well-established and even immutable, has undoubtedly been labouring under a great misapprehension for the list of new infectious diseases continues to grow. In July 1976 an epidemic appeared unexpectedly in Philadelphia. Legionnaires disease, a mystery respiratory condition that was eventually put down to bacteria adapted to live in air conditioning systems cooled down by water, was spread to the residents of a hotel attending a conference via the air conditioning in their rooms. AIDS was the next threat, which in a short period of time reached every corner of the planet. The World Health Organisation (WHO) calculated that by 1997 there would be more than 20 million humans infected with the HIV virus. In spite of the many pharmaceuticals that have been produced to combat it, the mortality rate continues to be high.§

Today the aggression of new viruses does not cease, many of them originating in Africa, such as Lasa fever (1969); the Ebola virus (1976); the Marburg virus (named after the German city of the same name where it produced 30 patients (7 fatal), contaminated by monkeys brought over from Uganda); Lyme's disease (caused by spirochetal bacteria and observed for the first time in the city of Lyme in the state of Connecticut on the Eastern coast of the United States).

One could also mention various new diseases like that caused by the "hanta" virus (named for the Hanta river in Korea, which killed several people in the south west of the United States in 1993), and the acute and severe respiratory syndrome (know by its initials as SARS, also called Asian pneumonia), which appeared in 2003, the evolution and consequences of which are still difficult to pinpoint.

There is no reason to think that we won't have new surprises to lament in the future.

§ *Note from Venezuelan American virologist José Esparza: Antiretroviral treatment, wherever it is used, is effective. That is evident at the individual level (the so-called Lazarus effect) as well as at the population level. In fact, the paradoxical effect is that in countries like the U.S., the number of people living with HIV is increasing (near 1.2 m) because people with HIV don't die as before and approximately 50,000 new HIV infections are added every year.*

32nd Paradox
Pain and power vs. Medicine and money

It is not necessarily a case of the first two being against the other two, rather that all four are intimately linked; at least this is the opinion offered by one of the most distinguished, albeit controversial, contemporary French intellectuals Jacques Attali in his book *L'Ordre Cannibale*.

His acerbic and hard criticisms, such as "half of health expenditure only serves to postpone death by a few weeks", or "eight tenths of humanity don't have any access to a medical clinic", cannot be brushed off in one stroke or completely forgotten; whether we like it or not, they are public denunciations that are based on facts.

I confess I admire the courage of Jean Bernard when he refers to his deep dislike of addressing matters concerning the antithetical pairing of medicine and money; it is a dislike that I share.

In reality, to the contrary of what many people might imagine (perhaps due to "exterior signs of wealth", such as a car, house or articles of expensive clothing), the number of medical professionals who amass a fortune through their work can be counted on one's fingers.

Suffice to say that there are very few truly rich doctors. Truly rich doctors' fortunes nearly always have a different origin than the practice of private medicine, and they have almost never, to my knowledge at least, economically benefited (as they surely would have been able to do) from patents for their important discoveries, which in other professions, trades and activities would have made their inventors millionaires.

33rd Paradox
Local medicine vs. Global medicine

Globalisation is all encompassing, an ocean of oil that does not cease to advance. We can no longer ignore or forget our neighbours' misfortunes, and what's more we live them in the very same moment in which they occur, which impedes us from resorting to evasive mechanisms and pleading ignorance. It used to be the case that we received the news much more passively due to the fact that we were informed of catastrophes or misfortunes hours, days, even months after they occurred (the time lapse depending on the era). In this generation we are able to watch major events as they happen; having been warned by telephone of the first attack, I will never forget watching the impact of the second plane against the other twin tower in New York "live" on television, on that fateful 11 September 2001.

In the context of medicine, this means that the developed and affluent, even opulent, countries of the North cannot put the poverty, misery and hunger of the South, and all of the painful consequences related to the health of these people, to one side. On the one hand, television brings full colour images – in these cases much more powerful than words – to the minds of the general public on a daily basis with great impact; on the other hand, we know all too well that political borders between countries or even large distances between continents do not offer protection from the great pandemics, as irrefutably proven by AIDS; they can appear without notice and with truly catastrophic results.

The medical profession, as a professional community, is aware that this is a reality that is no longer possible to ignore, and with the limited means within their reach they periodically make practical contributions (separately to and independently of the great work carried out by international bodies such as the World Health Organisation, and in our case, the Pan American Health Organisation, etc.). The contributions made are numerous and include, amongst other notable initiatives, "Doctors without Borders", "Doctors of the World", "International Medical Aid", etc., which are described by Oliver Weber in his book *French Doctors*.

I take this opportunity to highlight the extraordinary work carried out in the dermatology sector, to which I am sure you know I have been a privileged witness, by the International Foundation for Dermatology in East Africa (Moshi, Tanzania) under the presidency of Professors Alfred Kopf of New York University School of Medicine and Terence Ryan of the University of Oxford, in coordination with local work by the German dermatologist Henning Grossmann, to whom I wish to pay the sincere tribute that they deserve on this occasion. This sound work, which began in 1987, has permitted the provision of technical experts in dermatology to a good number of countries in the region, thereby reducing the incidences of contagious skin diseases especially in school populations.

34th Paradox
The truth vs. The partial truth

The Black Legend unjustly attributed such conduct to the Jesuits, but truth be told doctors can and must continually put this behaviour into practice. It boils down to the approach that their patients have the right to the truth, but only part of the truth. Let me explain: the doctor must attempt to understand how the patient thinks, and based on this understanding of his or her personality and character, must accordingly manage everything related to the diagnosis, prognosis and treatment of the patient's illness.

For example, I learned from my maternal uncle, Dr Martín Vegas, that a leprosy diagnosis cannot be given suddenly to the patient even if it is certain, for the shock, due to the terrible connotations of the suspected incurable, mutilating, contagious illness, can be of such magnitude that it makes the patient want to take their own life. Instead, if the patient is told of the possibility of this tragic diagnosis in stages, it is very possible that they will accept it without exhibiting the extreme behaviour determined by desperation. It is the same with many other diseases of sombre prognosis, for example cancer (in any of its forms or locations) or degenerative diseases of the brain (Alzheimer's disease, Parkinson's disease, etc.).

Personally I recall very well one of my first private patients when I returned to Caracas after specialising in the United States. My patient was a young man with neuritis of the ulnar nerve, stiffness in his little and ring fingers. It was fairly obvious that this was a typical case of tuberculoid leprosy and that I had to devise a strategy to explain the characteristics and foreseeable consequences of his disease carefully to the patient in private, which would not be easy. He was accompanied by his mother-in-law, married for only a few years with three very small children he had moved in with his in-laws and was working hard to maintain his family. It was hard to get the young man alone in order to be able to speak privately with him, but when I managed to do so I gradually introduced my suspected diagnosis. When I requested emphatically that any knowledge remain a secret between us, he flatly refused citing a religious basis for the trust between him and his wife, to whom he felt he had to communicate the truth of his affliction. Every time he refused to accept my conditions of keeping the matter secret, I asked him to think about it for another week. Only on the third occasion did he accept that I with my knowledge and experience as a doctor was best placed to interpret the facts, and he "yielded" to my "better judgement", although he was still not convinced. And so I treated him for several years until his complete cure, without his illness altering his family relationships, his work or contact with his wife and children. When on social occasions I casually bump into him surrounded by his children and grandchildren, and a successful executive of a solvent business, I am filled with happiness in the security that he does not remotely imagine how my determination saved not only his current prosperity, but also the stability of his marriage and family relationships. For unfortunately the terrible "stigma" of leprosy that has been so entrenched over the centuries does not even respect the firm religious convictions to which my patient turned.

35th Paradox
Hippocratic medicine vs. Iatrogenesis

When I refer to Hippocratic medicine I am fundamentally referring to the Latin phrase *primum non nocere* (first, do no harm), which is attributed to Hippocrates. This is the basis of professional medical practice and is the extreme opposite of iatrogenesis, that is to say, those illnesses that originate from the medical act.

The renowned controversialist Ivan Illich* begins his book *Limits to Medicine* by stating: "The medical establishment has become a major threat to health. The disabling impact of professional control over medicine has reached the proportions of an epidemic." (Illich, 1995: 1)

It is a serious problem and countries in possession of reliable statistics permit our understanding of the gravity of the situation; in the United States the use of synthetic pharmaceuticals, prescribed correctly or incorrectly, cause around 231,000 deaths every year.

In *Confessions of a Medical Heretic* by Dr Robert S. Mendelsohn, we encounter another terrifying statistic when he states that in the United States 2.4 million unnecessary surgical interventions are carried out every year, with a loss of 12,000 lives. (Mendelsohn, 1979: 49)

"Such *clinical iatrogenesis* includes not only the damage that doctors inflict with the intent of curing or of exploiting the patient, but also those other torts that result from the doctor's attempt to protect himself against the possibility of a suit for malpractice. Such attempts to avoid litigation and prosecution may now do more damage than any other iatrogenic stimulus." (Illich, 1995: 32–3)

It is possible that these are "alarmist" affirmations, but the role of the health authorities is to demonstrate that there is no substance in

---

* Ivan Illich (1926–2002), Philosopher of Austrian origin

such accusations, even if these are inflated or exaggerated figures there is a "grain of truth" in them that requires careful examination.[§]

Geoff Watts[*] highlights the work undertaken some years ago by a group of qualified doctors from Boston University Medical Centre, which followed 800 admitted patients. Within these 800 they confirmed 290 instances of iatrogenic disorders (illnesses that were not induced by nature or the behaviour of the patient, but instead by the medication or procedures prescribed by the doctors and in relation to the diagnosis and treatment of the ailment for which they were originally admitted to hospital); 76 of them suffered major complications and in 15 cases the iatrogenic disorder contributed to the cause of death. (Watts, 2006: 342)

Clarifying the meaning of a patient's illness is not the same with a hypochondriac patient as it is with an unconcerned and irresponsible patient, and doctors need to carefully ration out their explanation according to their relationship with the patient, which is based on their personality. At times they may emphasise certain details, and at other times play down their importance, all in order to achieve the same effect, which is that the patient understands the nature of their illness and faithfully follows the treatment prescribed to them. Success in professional practice depends in large part on the mental sharpness of the doctor in applying appropriate psychological reasoning and interpretation.

Mechanisms of iatrogenic origin can even extend to such vast areas as public health measures and preventative medicine. For example, the side effects of immunisation by the triple vaccine (DTaP – D for diphtheria, T for tetanus and aP for acellular pertussis, or whooping

§ *Alfred Kopf, MD: Another sinister act is for a physician to deliberately treat patients for diseases the patients do not have. See the Dr Farid Fata case (Today News: 2013)*

* Geoff Watts, medical writer and scientist of British origin

cough), the side effects include permanent organ damage, and are attributed to the pertussis component, perhaps without sustainable foundation, for which reason they have not been removed from the market. This has, however, caused an intense debate charged with accusations as exemplified in the book by Harris L. Coulter and Barbara Loe Fisher, *A Shot in the Dark: Why the P in the DPT vaccination may be hazardous to your child's health* (1991).

Once a doubt is introduced in the minds of the general public, it is difficult to remove it; such is the case with the possible link between autism and vaccinations that contain thiomersal (a toxic preservative for the central nervous system). Although dismissed by various scientific works, and even now that this chemical is no longer used in the majority of vaccines, such suspicion has awoken a negative attitude towards the vaccination of infants, which undoubtedly creates a problem: the risk of the contagious illnesses that vaccinations are intended to prevent, which is greater than that of the supposed illness that the vaccines could cause.

36th Paradox
Antibiotics and antivirals vs. Bacteria and mutating viruses

Ever since the discovery and first use of penicillin in 1941, the production of antibiotics, which are effective in treating illnesses caused by bacteria and protozoa, has been copious. However, we cannot possibly assume that this production is inexhaustible. Contradictorily, the mutagenic potential of bacteria and viruses does not have foreseeable limits, which in the long term may possibly lead to an unequal battle in which medicine slowly but surely loses ground. Similar reasoning can be applied to antiviral molecules against viruses.

Even in recent times, there has been no lack of controversy regarding well-established preventative medical procedures like vaccination, such as described in the aforementioned book by Harris L. Coulter and Barbara Loe Fisher, *A Shot in the Dark: Why the P in the DPT vaccination may be hazardous to your child's health,* which was specifically intended to warn parents of the potential danger of the whooping cough vaccine.

As discussed in the previous paradox, this situation has provoked an infinite number of writings and even formal organisations dedicated to informing the general public of the possible risks of vaccination. Such controversy has planted doubt in parent's minds and has complicated the preventative action of paediatricians who must continually evaluate the benefits of immunisation versus the supposed risks; risks that even if proven would still be very limited.

37th Paradox
Curative medicine vs. Hygiene

While these may be different disciplines, they are often closely linked. This is especially due to the fact that the undeniable influence of hygiene in maintaining good health has been irrefutably established.

As John Pickstone[*] rightly said: "We often think of medicine as a progress that flows through recent history. Medicine is part of a complex interaction in economic and political history. Its future, as well as its past, in the 'second' and 'third world', as well as in the West, will depend on the changing models of wealth and power."

It is impossible to disagree with Laurie Garrett[†] in her book, *Betrayal of Trust*: ". . . the basic factors essential to a population's health are ancient and non-technological: clean water; plentiful, nutritious uncontaminated food; decent housing; appropriate water and waste disposal; correct social and medical control of epidemics; widespread – or universal – access to maternal and child health-care; clean air; knowledge of personal health needs administered to a population sufficiently educated to be able to comprehend and use the information in their daily lives; and, finally, a health-care system that follows the primary maxim of medicine – do no harm." (Garrett, 2001: 12)

There will always be dissent over the relative importance of these two factors in the benefits that are generally accepted in the health sector; in many respects they are both supplementary and inextricable.

[*] John Pickstone, 1944–2014, physiologist and historian of English science at the University of Manchester
[†] Laurie Garrett, American scientific journalist and writer

38th Paradox
Accurate diagnosis vs. Effective treatment

For centuries medicine made slow but continuous progress and during this time doctors accumulated invaluable information about the natural history of diseases, which is very useful in establishing a bad prognosis, but of little practical interest for the patient who is exclusively interested in a curative treatment for their illness.

With reference to the discovery of circulation by William Harvey (1578–1657), it is said that a man as erudite as Thomas Jefferson (1743–1826) said to Edward Jenner (1749–1823) that it was, "a beautiful addition to our knowledge of the animal economy, but on a review of the practice of medicine before and since that epoch, I do not see any great amelioration which has been derived from that discovery." (Jefferson cited in Lachlan, 2010)

This situation can be applied to other discoveries in medicine (with the notable exception of vaccines and serum treatments) up until the advent of sulphonamides and antibiotics at the end of the first half of the twentieth century.

And so, after so many paradoxes we have an equation without un-knowns: public health = global prevention.

It is no longer possible to strive for a public health programme that only benefits citizens in isolated and protected dwellings; towns, cities, states, nations, regions and continents must benefit too. Modern transport means are swift, and, as we are well aware, a contagious disease in full incubation period can be transported to the most distant extremes of the Earth in a matter of a few hours. In a way, the recent AIDS epidemic has been enlightening in the fact that there exists no valid way of establishing an efficient "quarantine" against a scourge of this nature.

I personally observed the turning point for the leaders of worldwide medicine, in my case the most renowned lecturers and researchers in the field of dermatology who I would visit for meetings at the American Academy of Dermatology. They would listen patiently to my pleas for their support of any effort to help the development of specialisms in developing countries – like those in Africa and certain parts of Latin America – with a focus upon the importance of the tropical diseases that affected their inhabitants, but their patience was accompanied by a look that clearly said: it's not my problem, I don't have anything to do with this. Years later, the appearance of AIDS changed their attitude diametrically; as it became evident that diseases, at least many of them, do not abide by climates or borders. That change was subsequently clearly expressed by the creation of the International Foundation for Dermatology and its work in East Africa (Tanzania).

39th Paradox
Fashions in medicine vs. Immutable truths

Lay people always have and always will interfere in medical matters. Nor is there a shortage of sceptics who believe they have the last word on lifestyle. For example: "Early to rise and early to bed makes a man healthy, wealthy, and dead", James Thurber.* Or, those who believe doctors should listen to the advice that they have no qualms in recommending or inflicting on others. For example: "Physician, heal thyself!"

Although the public may not notice it, over a certain transitional period, fashion overwhelmingly affects and penetrates medical practice. When I began my medical studies, bloodletting, leeches and colon cleansing were medical practices of the past, yet tonsillectomies (accompanied or not by adenoidectomies), indiscriminate appendectomies, artificial pneumothorax, electroshocks and scarification and cupping were not. Other fashions have been implemented since then, and after a period of popularity these too will certainly gradually die out before they disappear into total oblivion.

* James Thurber (1894–1961), American writer and cartoonist

40th Paradox
The battle against illness vs. The battle against death

Given that many illnesses have a fatal prognosis (i.e. will end in death), the first is frequently associated with the second, although of course the majority of cases of illness do not result in death. However, it should be remembered that James C. Riley* has encouraged the concept of a synergy that he refers to as "insult accumulation" (Riley, 1989: 47). We know that these days the majority of episodes of illness do not lead to death, as they probably didn't in the past either. But according to Riley, each episode of illness followed by recuperation leaves a certain residue (or scar) of harm or weakness in the organism. Further episodes have a cumulative effect that eventually leads to the patient's death. And so the hypothesis is reached that every new insult to their health leaves the individual more susceptible to illness in the future. All of this leads him to postulate that those people who have enjoyed good health at the beginning of their lives will live longer and with greater vigour. Recent generations of doctors have been trained for an endless and unapologetic battle against the natural and inevitable fact of every living being's death which is, in a significant number of cases, attributed to the failure of appropriate and efficient medical care. It is therefore both natural and understandable that the general public adopts a similar point of view and won't accept the harsh reality of ageing, of the degenerative diseases that accompany it, and finally, of death, as the natural termination of our lifecycle.

The great irony of modern medicine is that these days geriatrics, one of the least valued specialisms, occupies the majority of hospital beds. The central problem of geriatrics as a medical specialism is

* James C. Riley, demography historian at the University of Indiana

recognising the fact that at the end of the day we human beings are mortal and necessarily must die from some terminal event, which remains, as it has been throughout history, by its very nature uncertain as far as understanding and handling it is concerned.

Perhaps the best health strategy is to try to maintain the body in a good state, both physically and mentally, until shortly before death. With this strategy, the paradox comes from the fact that it is highly probable that in increasing the life expectancy of the patient, the possibility of developing degenerative diseases and mental incapacity is increased. "How many people would thank medicine for a similar gift?"

41st Paradox

Waste vs. Rationalisation in the use of medical equipment

The high cost of modern apparatus in imaging, which includes tomographs and magnetic resonance, and radiography equipment, leads us to believe that some rationalisation should be applied in their acquisition and use. If this is the case in the public sector, it is also advisable in the private sector, whenever reaching a partnership agreement between clinics and private hospitals is feasible. In order to make that "rationality" more convincing, our academic colleague Ladimiro Espinoza compared the costs of some of the more expensive pieces of equipment with what could be done in other operational areas of those institutions if funds were utilised in a different direction.

We reach the conclusion that in this era of continual new technological advances, specialists behave like children with new toys, and will always find convincing arguments to justify numerous investments in apparatus, which if put to better use could benefit citizens and, at times, even regions or countries. On the other hand we cannot discount the potential temptation to indiscriminately order tests in order to recoup the high costs incurred (we would hope that no such temptation exists with treatments).

A similar situation occurs with certain new pharmaceuticals, which can incur extremely elevated costs due in part to the investment in research required to discover and develop them; this coupled with a limited market serves as justification for their inaccessible prices.

42nd Paradox
Leisure time vs. Reflection time

It is said, perhaps with some reason, that the notable contributions to universal culture made by the Greeks and the Hellenistic civilisation are due in part to the slave system prevalent during that period, as this permitted citizens of various city-states to excuse themselves from all domestic activity (which was relegated to the slaves) and thereby have the time to meditate, think, reason, discuss and write.

With the advent of machines, which has diminished or nullified the importance of physical force (in which men have the advantage over women), the differences between the sexes in intellectual work have become hazy or have completely disappeared. Furthermore, with the invention of the computer, the human brain (masculine or feminine) has been able to trust many analytical tasks to machines, and concentrate on synthesis, which seems to be the superior function of this organ.

There are those who have suggested that the extreme temperatures of hot tropical countries are a hindrance to fruitful intellectual work; if there is any truth in this, it is possible that air conditioning may liberate the intellectual potential of inhabitants of that broad geographic sector of the planet.

The theory that associates leisure (here I refer to the leisure of routine and strenuous activity) with intellectual activity undoubtedly has its merits, and a cursory reading of the biographies of great thinkers demonstrates that they had the time, along with a certain economic autonomy, to think. Which is what a man of sharp mind like the publicist Carlos Eduardo Frías captured perfectly when he stated that in order to be productive, intellectually speaking, one had to, "buy the freedom to think". Reflecting on the creativity of the Scottish, somebody pointed out that the severity of the winter climate meant that for many months they were unable to do anything other than sit in front of the fire-place and "knit socks", which certainly gave them time to think. Abraham Flexner (1866–1959), educator, and the person who has had most influence on all related to contemporary medical education (The Flexner Report), had no doubt about this and expressed it very clearly by tirelessly, and with great conviction, supporting the full-time teacher system in university faculties of medicine, believing that teachers contracted thus would be capable of, "dedicating their time and energy to careful study and experimentation, whilst they read in many languages, conversed, discussed, and reflected unhurriedly ... as the doctor grappled with the most complicated mechanism; the human body".

This system either eliminates or limits the potential ambition of a successful doctor in private practice from attempting to establish a veritable industry with their knowledge, as it sets rather inflexible rates and time constraints for that type of professional practice. Until only recently such extremes existed: I recall a colleague who bragged about the long queues of patients every day who would wait until the early hours of the morning for a consultation with him. Such excess an of "routine" work certainly does not induce creative thought.

One of the most distinguished mathematicians of our times said as much to me in Cambridge, where he was a neighbour of the house in which I was staying. When answering a half-acid, half-humorous observation on my part, he replied very seriously referring to the time that he would spend in his garden playing with his ferret: "Remember that the University pays me to think ... and it is on those occasions that I think best."

This is what the effect and consequences of special working considerations for teachers should be, like for example the "sabbatical year", which, when effectively and reasonably employed, should result in measurable intellectual progress and productivity amongst university teachers, something that is still to be proven in our environment.

43rd Paradox
Cardiopulmonary death vs. Brain death

With advances in resuscitation techniques and the possibility of vital organ transplants, this issue began to be seriously contemplated from the 1960s onwards. In the past, people had an understandable apprehension that "by error of a definitive and irreversible death diagnosis they could be 'buried alive'". Given that the accepted definition of death has changed from the suspension of heart beats and respiration (which with suitable machines can be maintained artificially) to that of brain death, which is determined by two successive flat (i.e. without activity) electroencephalographs, these days in consideration of the possibility of recovering from a brain coma, people are more concerned about the possibility of being "dismembered" (in the sense of losing a vital organ) before the heart and lungs have stopped functioning.

44th Paradox
Health balance: Diet vs. Lifestyle vs. Environment

As is the case with so many other apparent paradoxes, this one looks at three factors that compete and collaborate in intricate ways for the good health of the individual.

It is well known that the health expectancy of people who live in the rich and industrialised countries of the North is much higher than that of the poor who live in the South.§ In the North there is much exploitation of ideas (with little scientific basis) that promise to stop or even reverse ageing in order to restore a lost physical beauty, all with clear economic success for the physicians who carry them out.

The truth is that the "social appetite" for health has no known limits. This is summed up in the famous *dictum* made by the British politician Enoch Powell (1912–98) when he was Health Minister: "there is virtually no limit to the amount of medical care an individual is capable of absorbing." (Powell cited in Annas, 1998: 74)

§ *Note from the author in response to a request from Alfred Kopf, MD for clarification of the meaning of "North" and "South": For many years, even centuries, people took for granted that all of the developed countries were in the Northern part of the world (North of the Equator), and that the South meant under development. At present this rule has the exception of Australia and New Zealand (and perhaps South Africa). By chance I suppose this applies as well to the United States (at least prior to the American Civil War).*

45th Paradox
The history of medicine vs. The history of human society's efforts to control health problems and disease

In truth this is not a paradox but rather two different viewpoints that must integrate, for when all is said and done they have identical objectives. The current tendency to focus on the history of medicine from the point of view of the doctor, such as in the work of Henry E. Sigerist[*] and Roy Porter,[†] constitutes a healthy change of attitude and a suitable orientation as "it is the patient, or better still the healthy or unwell man, who is the object of all of the doctor's actions."

[*] Henry E. Sigerist (1891–1957), French doctor and medical historian
[†] Roy Porter (1946–2002), British medical historian

46th Paradox
The discredit of the doctor: Craftsman vs. Technologist

One of the hardest and most implacable critics of contemporary medicine, Ivan Illich (1926–2002) said, "With the transformation of the doctor from an artisan exercising a skill on personally known individuals into a technician applying scientific rules to classes of patients, malpractice acquired an anonymous, almost respectable status." (Illich, 1975: 24)

Medicine is therefore a complicated blend for it contains undeniably desirable ingredients of both craft and technology, which we doctors prefer to classify as art and science, although in truth they are both valid, mutually complementary bases that serve as a foundation for medicine.

47th Paradox
Medical progress vs. Socio-economic progress

We should be under no illusion that progress and advancement in the field of public health, or even in private medical practice, can be achieved in isolation. The environment in which medicine operates makes it a more or less effective activity. Socio-political and cultural context is crucial, as much for permitting medicine to develop institutionally as for achieving its successful transplantation in places where it has not spontaneously emerged.

One of the reasons for the apparent triumph of Western civilisation over other contemporary cultures, such as Japanese, Chinese and Hindu cultures, lies in the effectiveness of its medicine. All initial contacts between Western medicine and its potential rivals undoubtedly demonstrate the superiority of its scientifically orientated results.

48th Paradox
Collaboration with the pharmaceutical industry vs. Conflict of interests with the medical profession

The enormous growth of the pharmaceutical industry has always relied upon a close working relationship with the medical class. This is especially the case with university lecturers, that is to say, the academic sector of the profession in relation to the evaluation of the effectiveness of new pharmaceuticals.

Given the magnitude of the pharmaceutical industry and the costs involved in developing a new drug (estimated to be between 300 and 600 million dollars, some analysts take it to a billion or more) and including therapeutic tests in clinical trials, it is easy to imagine the significant amounts invested in this sector which is so important to the future commercialisation of a new medicine. The eventual approval of the health authorities depends in large part on these evaluations, on the methodology utilised, as well as the seriousness and good reputation of the doctors who carry out the evaluation and of the institutions for which they work. In the United States it is estimated that for every day of delay in the FDA's (Food and Drug Administration) approval process, the manufacturer loses an average of 1.3 million dollars.

It is well known that these types of study are financially dependent on the generosity and very well defined interest of the pharmaceutical industry, with the industry estimated to provide 70% of the funds for medical clinical trials. The improper promotion of some pharmaceutical products is supported by numerous publications of work that is undeserving, or worse still unknown or containing rigged information.

This is an area that must be continually monitored by the medical profession in order to avoid excesses, abuses and deviations in a field in which the existence of evident economic incentives can generate a broad range of acts that are, in essence, corrupt. The ethical foundations of placebo-controlled trials have been seriously questioned. An interpretation of the Helsinki declaration appears to indicate that placebo controlled trials are unethical, with the statement: "In any medical study every patient, including those in a control group, if there is one, should be guaranteed access to the best proven diagnostic and therapeutic method of treatment available." (Botbol-Baum, 2000: 238–45)

When we carry out one of these trials we know *a priori* that half of the cases is receiving a placebo, i.e. without any therapeutic value, and are therefore not being treated with a pharmaceutical that can cure or improve their illness (although we are intentionally unable to identify with any certainty which cases these are); a problem of insoluble ethical order which has been questioned with compelling arguments, as "there is no circumstance under which an effective treatment may be withheld."

Given that they only prove significant differences with the placebo and there is no improvement over the baseline, there are those who believe that placebo-controlled trials are unnecessary.

The relationship between the pharmaceutical industry (and even manufacturers of medical and hospital equipment) and doctors is essential to the progress of medicine, but it can generate conflicts of interest and must be managed with integrity and transparency.

In an anecdotal and personal capacity I recall the visit of a patient who was a top executive in the Venezuelan pharmaceutical industry. He expressed, with a certain degree of conviction, his complaints about the medical profession, who in addition to the same old contributions to their congresses, seminars, conferences and even events of an educational character, proposed, and at times even demanded funds to construct sporting facilities (for example swimming pools) in the headquarters of medical schools at a national level. I stared at him and replied: "Apart from those donations to scientific meetings in which you have a vested interest in raising awareness of your products, tell me truthfully, what you have done for the scientific progress of medicine in Venezuela." This conversation led to the Fundación Vargas initiative, which played an important role in clinical research but which later disappeared without valid reason, suffering the fate of those institutions that die out from wear and tear or anachronism.

49th Paradox

Gender differences: Male doctors vs. Female doctors

These days when many Faculties of Medicine have an equal number of students of both sexes, sometimes even more females than males, it is hard to believe that until the end of the nineteenth century women were prohibited from studying our profession.

It was the same with all professional university degrees, a little over a century ago it was not conceived of for women to study and then practise a liberal profession. This was one of the goals demanded by the feminist movement, which was achieved with much effort over a period of many years. Although antiquity offers an abundance of examples of notable women who practised as healers and midwives, many of them paid highly for their supposed audacity and were the object of merciless persecutions and accused, often unjustly, of being witches and sorcerers, ending up burned alive at the stake.

Eventually *demonomania* was "medicalised" and its supposed manifestations came to be considered as symptoms of mental illnesses (hysteria, etc.).

The first woman to obtain a medical university degree was Dorotea Christiane Exleben-Leporin (1715–62), the daughter of a local doctor from the small Prussian town of Quedlinburg. In 1740 she asked permission from the King of Prussia, Frederick the Great, to read medical studies at the University of Halle, and after many difficulties (marriage, motherhood, etc.) finally obtained her degree in 1754. This turned out to be a mere accident, an isolated case in Europe, as the ensuing consequences did not happen for many years.

The arguments used to impede women from practising medicine were supposedly specific to their gender; arguments lacking weight, such as mental and physical incapacity due to menstruation, lack of physical strength, incapacity caused by pregnancy and breastfeeding, mental inferiority due to a smaller brain, and the habitual complaint that medical work would rob the woman of her femininity.

The first woman to receive a medical doctorate in the English-speaking world was the North American Elizabeth Blackwell (1821–1910), who received her degree from Geneva College in the State of New York in 1849.

However, for Venezuelans it is interesting to highlight the achievements of Dr James Miranda Barry (1795–1865), who in 1812 graduated in medicine from the University of Edinburgh, precisely in the period of that School of Medicine's greatest fame (it was there that the great Venezuelan doctor José María Vargas (1786–1854) achieved the almost simultaneous perfection of his medical and basic science studies). Dr James Miranda Barry had an outstanding professional career as a military doctor in different British colonies, introducing important reforms in the service and rose up to the final rank of general inspector (equivalent to that of a general); it was only when she died that her feminine gender become known.

There is wide evidence of a close relationship with General Francisco Miranda (1750–1816), the forefather of Latin American independence, who is credited in her doctorate thesis dedication. Ruth Bowden* deepened this relationship further by attributing the paternity of Barry to Miranda. This was captured in the novel *James Miranda Barry* written by Patricia Duncker (1951–) and published in 1999.

Even in my days as a student of medicine when there already existed a small group of female medical students, I recall the comments of my loved and admired professor of anatomy José Izquierdo who half

* Ruth Bowden (1915–2001), British doctor and professor of Anatomy at the School of Medicine of the Royal Free Hospital in London

jokingly told the female students that they didn't go to medical school to "warm the seats", referring directly to the fact that he believed that after graduation many of them (having used up a "quota" of limited access to medical studies), would marry, have children and abandon medical practice.

The tendency at a worldwide level is that enrolment in medical schools by both sexes behaves much like that of the general population, with recent WHO figures putting medical school graduation at 52% men and 48% women.

The total number of doctors in the United States is estimated to be 836,156 of which 205,903 are women, or 24.6% (for the year 2001). This figure will certainly increase progressively over the years to reach equality between the sexes, something that is already observed in the rank of Assistant Professor in Faculties of Medicine, where women already occupy 50.1% of the available positions (compared with 10.7% in the role of full professor.)

This is therefore a paradox of the past which has found its correction with time, as there is nobody who currently advocates discrimination against women studying and practising medicine, not even in fundamentalist Muslim countries like Iran. When we visited this country in 2001 we found a large number of girls (with their heads covered by black headscarves and chador) studying medicine and actively working in all hospitals.

50th Paradox
The rise vs. The fall of medicine

Paraphrasing the British writer and historian Edward Gibbon (1737–94) in his classic book of five volumes *The History of the Decline and Fall of the Roman Empire* (1776 to 1788), the British medical writer James Le Fanu published a book of great interest, as already mentioned, in which he offers an intelligent analysis of the great achievements of medicine in the years that followed the Second World War. These include some great victories such as those against smallpox, diphtheria and polio, and the discovery of medication to control the progress of Parkinson's disease, rheumatoid arthritis and schizophrenia, and also open-heart surgery, organ transplants and test tube babies. Three decades later such spectacular advances no longer occur, and the promises of medical social theories, genetics and statistical deductions have not produced the results that were hoped for.

The "Twelve Definitive Moments" of recent medical innovation are identified as the discoveries of penicillin, cortisone, smoking identified as the cause of lung cancer, chlorpromazine, intensive care, open-heart surgery, hip replacement, kidney transplant, control of high blood pressure (and prevention of strokes), cure of childhood cancer, test tube babies, and the importance of Helicobacter. (Le Fanu, 2011: 3)

Aside from these definitive moments, Le Fanu shows very little optimism that molecular biology truly drives us, as many analysts believe, to more rational forms of treatment or even the prevention of common illnesses.§

§ *Alfred Kopf, MD: This discussion seems a little one-sided as a "downer" on recent advancements in medicine. One example in my field of melanoma is the truly remarkable development of tailored medicaments based on newer understanding of the basic process of the melanoma cell and the immunologic response to this*

The North American doctor William B. Schwartz* offered a contrasting opinion in his book *Life without Disease: The Pursuit of Medical Utopia* and his optimism about the potential of molecular biology and genetics was shared by Sir John Maddox† in *What Remains to be Discovered.*

cancer, which is the background for the development of new drugs emerging today. And, how about the drugs for HIV infection – most AIDS patients now have long lives with continued viral suppression. My conclusion is that medicine is improving at a much faster pace compared to the past.

* William B. Schwartz (1923–2009), American nephrologist
† Sir John Maddox (1925–2009), British scientist, editor of the influential journal *Nature* for 12 years

51st Paradox
Expected death vs. Premature death

The "years of potential life lost" concept (YPLL) is an important gauge, which taking into account its economic importance must be given the priority that it deserves by medical care strategies.

Indeed all public health organisation strategies throughout the world, such as those noted by Dr Rómulo Orta Cabrera in his work in Venezuela, must give this gauge the importance it deserves. It reveals the loss of hundreds of thousands of lives (in Venezuela the rate increased from 474,819 in 1985 to 982,568 in 1995), "however, in the year 2000, the Ministry of Health and Social Development programmes focused on child and maternal health and the distribution of contraceptives."

52nd Paradox
The best medical care vs. Ordinary medical care

It is widely believed that there exists a continually expanding breach between the best medical care available and routine, common or ordinary medical care.

This is medicine's eternal dilemma. Medical services have a cost, indeed one that increases with each day that passes, and although throughout history doctors as individuals have always tried, using the most diverse means possible, to bring medical attention to the most humble, poor and those who lack the economic means to pay for those services, they are always playing catch-up. It is no longer possible to pretend that such social reality is the responsibility of just the individual rather than the responsibility of society as a whole.

Although social security programmes are intended to close the breach between the haves and the have-nots, and although in some developed countries (above all Northern European countries) the quality of medical services amongst those who pay additionally for private services and those available for free to the general public are approximately the same level, there is always a favourable difference for those who have the economic means to pay for private medicine. Compare the National Health Service waiting lists for surgical intervention in Great Britain with the speed with which those who have the means to pay for private insurance or direct payment of hospital and doctors' fees are able to proceed.

53rd Paradox
The eternal conflict: Ontologists vs. Physiologists

Since time immemorial the history of medicine has been witness to a deep philosophical discrepancy between those who believe illness is its own entity that acts autonomously (ontologists), and those who think, by contrast, that the illness and ill person form an inseparable unit and that therefore the concept of illness cannot exist in isolation from the ill person (physiologists). Interestingly, these two ideas have swung back and forth like a pendulum throughout the centuries, at least in the history of Western medicine, with one or the other tendency being favoured at different periods.

In reality the issue is significantly more complex, the concept of illness has evolved with time and there exist various interpretative models. The most well known are:

1 Nosological and reactivist ontologism:
As previously explained, this maintains that illness is something that is separate from the individual. The illness attacks the individual, penetrates them, makes them ill, and eventually ends their life. Reactivism understands illness as the reaction of the organism.

2 Holistic and reductionist models:
The holistic understands illness as a global reaction, that it is to say something that affects the body as well as the mind. Reductionist models believe that illness has a limited and precise localisation, with anatomical or functional alteration. On the other hand when the focus is on the illness this is known as:

    a Histopathological model
    b Pathophysiological model
    c Etiopathogenic model

And when the subject is incorporated with the concept of illness, the following arise:

        a Characterological model
        b Psychosomatic model
        c Psychoanalytic model
        d Psychosocial model
        e Anthropological model

In short, it would be necessary to combine these and other factors in order to thoroughly understand the illness acting upon the human being.

54th Paradox
Quality of medicine: A technical problem vs. A cultural issue

Known critics of North American medicine believe that the main problem that it confronts is a matter of culture, and not technology as is frequently claimed without looking at the case in any depth.

I recall that this was the case some years ago in the state of Táchira, Venezuela, where severely ill children were hospitalised for malnutrition (a syndrome similar to "kwashiorkor" in South Africa, which occurs in children fed exclusively on corn, a grain that is deficient in essential amino acids, lysine and tryptophan).

It was established that their poor nutrition did not result from the most obvious factor, which was the poverty of the population, but was instead a cultural problem as the mothers were accustomed to feeding their infants exclusively with a type of corn drink called "atole". This situation clearly explains the epidemiology of this particular illness, and highlights the possibility of controlling and curing it with good health education programmes.

Some decades ago, the Institute of Nutrition of Central America (INCAP) designed a corn flour fortified with fishmeal, etc. (called "Incaparina"), in order to resolve a problem of a similar nature in Guatemala. The Rockefeller Foundation in Cali, Colombia used genetic manipulation to produce a corn hybrid containing a sufficient quantity of lysine and tryptophan called Maíz Opaco 2. Neither of these two strategies employed to impersonate common corn with something similar converted into a "complete food" had the definitive success that was hoped for, as overcoming cultural barriers is often much more difficult than anticipated.

55th Paradox

The contribution of doctors to medicine vs. Doctors' contributions to other branches of the cultural universe

Society clearly expects doctors to be responsible for contributions, innovations, research, discoveries and inventions in the field in which they have trained. However, we have already seen the notable importance of those medical discoveries or attention to medicine made by non-medical scientists (Pasteur, Röntgen, Curie, etc.).

From their establishment in the Middle Ages and through the centuries that ensued, after the initial degree in the arts, universities only offered three opportunities for postgraduate study: theology, medicine and law. Bearing this in mind, it is easy to assume that those people interested in the sciences studied medicine.

Simply listing only those medicine graduates that stood out in other fields of knowledge would fill a book, like in effect the book already published by T. K. Monro,* which includes a list of more than 500 people. Some were capable of actively practising medicine and made important contributions to other disciplines; others, having studied medicine, dedicated themselves to other activities where they achieved fame and universal prestige. However, it is possible that their medical studies exerted an abiding influence on their thinking and later work. It is also logical to suppose that there will also have been doctors who were distinguished by activities that were undesirable or illicit.

For reasons of space we will limit ourselves to mentioning only the most famous in the first category.

SCIENCES: Nicolaus Copernicus (1473–1543), Robert Boyle (1627–91), Robert Brown (1773–1858), Carl Linnaeus (1708–78).

* T. K. Monro (1865–1958), Scottish doctor, professor at the University of Glasgow

LITERATURE: François Rabelais (1494–1553), John Keats (1795–1821), Oliver Wendell Holmes (1809–1894), Axel Munthe (1857–1949), Sir Arthur Conan Doyle (1859–1930), Anton Pavlovich Chekhov (1860–1904), William Somerset Maugham (1874–1965), Sir Geoffrey Langdon Keynes (1887–1982), Archibald Joseph Cronin (1896–1981).

CHURCH: 29 saints and medical martyrs. The most well-known are Saint Luke (the Evangelist), the martyrs Saints Cosmas and Damian (303 AD), and Saint Pantaleon (305 AD). There was even a Pope who was a doctor, Petrus Julianus (1215–1277), professor of medicine in Sienna, and elected Pope John XXI in 1276.

MISSIONARIES AND EXPLORERS: David Livingstone (1813–73) and Albert Schweitzer (1875–1965).

PHILOSOPHY: Maimonides or Moshe ben Maimon (1135–1204), John Locke (1632–1704), William James (1842–1910).

MUSIC: Alexander Porfiryevich Borodin (1833–87).

POLITICS: Jean Paul Marat (1743–1793), Rudolf Virchow (1821–1902), Georges Benjamin Clemenceau (1841–1929), Sun Yat-sen (1866–1925).

There even existed a deified doctor, Imhotep (2850 BC), in Ancient Egypt.

Amongst the famous students of medicine who didn't end up graduating and practising medicine are Galileo Galilei (1564–1642), Johann Wolfgang von Goethe (1749–1832), Sir Humphry Davy (1778–1829), Hector Berlioz (1803–69), Charles Robert Darwin (1809–82), Sir Francis Galton (1822–1911) and Bertolt Brecht (1898–1956).

In Venezuela we can recall, amongst many others, José María Vargas and Jaime Lusinchi (in politics), Lisandro Alvarado (essayist), Arístides Rojas (historian), Blas Bruni Celli (historian) and Francisco José Herrera Luque (novelist).

56th Paradox

The right of invalids and the infirm to receive help vs. The right of the doctor to treat them

Experimentation on humans, and all things related to it, has for centuries been a matter of great interest to both doctors and the general public alike. There are many different suggested models in human experimentation, such as the golden rule model (by James Gregory in 1804), "Never carry out an experiment on anyone that you would not wish to have done on yourself, or on your dearest ones, if you or they were in the same situation as your patients"; the laboratory model (Claude Bernard in 1865); the public health/military medicine model (Walter Reed in 1900) and the patient model (Albert Moll in 1902).

In his book on medical ethics *Ärztliche Ethik*, published in 1902, the German doctor Albert Moll (1862–1939) develops the idea that there exist two reciprocal rights. After studying more than 600 cases he proposed the following moral principles (of the "patient as a model") to regulate medical experimentation on humans:

1   Every experiment must maximise potential benefits and minimise risk.
2   The risk must be weighed in consideration of the medical benefit rather than the scientific benefit.
3   Every possible laboratory test and tests on animals must be carried out before experimentation on humans.
4   Candidates must give their informed consent.
5   Written consent must be solicited and obtained before any relatively invasive procedures.
6   The written consent itself does not become an unduly risky experiment in ethics, nor does the consent justify the repetition of experiments.

7 There are certain groups of people who are inappropri
ate for experimentation, for example the dying, those
awaiting the death penalty, various categories of "institutionalised" people, and children. The protection of
the dying is a recurring preoccupation, suggesting that
exploitation of this group used to be fairly frequent.

8 Experimental results must be investigated with great
veracity.

9 Results of investigations must be adequately published.
Moll was concerned about the monopolistic power of
the editors of science magazines.

10 Experiments must always be carried out by competent
groups with clearly defined responsibilities.

This is basically the model that is currently adopted, fuelled to a
certain extent by knowledge of the horrors of human experimentation
during the Nazi regime in Germany, which were revealed by the Nurem-
berg trials (1946).

In the 1960s both the British Medical Association (1963) and
the American Medical Association (1966) published their respective
guidelines on human experimentation.

In 1964 the World Medical Association produced the Helsinki
Declaration (this was revised in 1975), placing the model of the patient
in its rightful place: "The health of my patient will be my first consideration." "While the primary purpose of medical research is to generate
new knowledge, this goal can never take precedence over the rights
and interests of individual research subjects."

57th Paradox
Current medical knowledge vs. Medical knowledge acquired at medical school

With the explosive growth of scientific knowledge, particularly medical knowledge, keeping doctors up to date in practice has become vital as the fact that they have studied medicine, graduated and obtained a licence to practise at a given moment is no longer enough. Within a few years some of the knowledge acquired in the classrooms and hospitals of medical faculties is already obsolete, and scientific and medical trade bodies should ensure that all of their associates keep their knowledge current. In the past, this interest in renewing knowledge was left to the discretion of each professional; the most successful in practice were nearly always those who combined teaching with the practice of medicine, those who held appointments in public university hospitals, those who published work, those who attended conferences and scientific meetings and those who were recognised by and formed part of the most prestigious scientific associations. However, these days this is not enough, and regulatory bodies in the most advanced countries have introduced clear rules that doctors must follow in order to maintain their professional practice licences. Some of these rules are "voluntary" but in practice it is very difficult for physicians who do not observe them to remain active.

In the United States professional organisations like the American Medical Association, the American College of Physicians, the American College of Surgeons and the "boards" of different specialisms have developed a great variety of "continued medical education" programmes in order to facilitate the acquisition of new knowledge and keep their associates up to date on every branch of medicine.

"Recertification" is already an accepted fact and something that will undoubtedly be gradually enforced in other countries. Online multimedia programmes permit doctors to study from their homes and surgeries, on the days and times that suit them best.

58th Paradox
Scientific controversies are resolved by:
Compelling arguments vs. Procedure vs. Natural death vs.
Resolution by negotiation

Medical controversies are interrelated with scientific controversies, especially biological ones. For this reason, it must be mentioned, albeit very briefly, that there is an inscrutable difference in the way in which these problems that deeply affect contemporary society are resolved.

Tom L. Beauchamp* looks at this topic in his chapter "Ethical Theory and the Problem of Closure" in the book *Scientific Controversies*.

This is a complex philosophical problem for which different eras and cultures have found diverse solutions.

The first type of resolution is reached when a "correct" opinion is formed; the second is achieved via arbitration procedures (legal for example); the third when interest in a certain subject simply declines; and the fourth via a negotiated compromise.

Conflict resolution in negotiation in many areas including science, medicine etc., is typical of contemporary North American society, where an acceptable solution between two extreme opposites is generally found. Conversely, for those countries that have adopted communism the controversy would always end via the first method, as repeatedly occurred in the former Soviet Union.

* Tom L. Beauchamp (1939–), American philosopher

59th Paradox

Biomedical research: Duty of the State vs. Philanthropic institutions' contributions

What today's world teaches us with complete clarity is that when society makes health problems one of its first priorities, it must find a suitable and practical way for public and private sectors to work together. The United States has clearly succeeded in using negotiation as the appropriate method for resolving conflicts, even in science where at first glance the truth is absolute and discussion is not permitted.

The debt that US medical development and its evident worldwide consequences owe to private philanthropy is of great importance.

The great "barons" and billionaires of American industry, specifically John D. Rockefeller* and Andrew Carnegie† shared an ethical view of the enormous fortunes that their work, wisdom and the explosive economic development of their country allowed them to accumulate. At the end of their lives they felt it necessary to reinvest a considerable amount of the money they had amassed into works of an enduring social interest. This saw the birth of the great foundations that carry their names, which are undoubtedly good reason for "immortalising" them in the memory of the societies that benefit from their actions. Those new institutions very quickly found that the best advantage that they could offer to society would be to support the development of the health sector. This was also the origin of the Wellcome Trust, established in 1903 by the pharmacist Sir Henry Wellcome, a British citizen of American heritage; given that the origins of his fortune lay in the nascent pharmaceutical industry, it was logical that he would be inextricably bound to medicine.

The most moving and enlightening story that I have heard on this

* John D. Rockefeller (1839–1937), American oil entrepreneur who founded Standard Oil. † Andrew Carnegie (1835–1919) Scottish-American steel tycoon.

matter relates to how John D. Rockefeller became interested in the development of medical studies and research as part of his philanthropic projects. According to this version, Rockefeller consulted with a religious friend who had just finished reading the medical textbook by Sir William Osler. This was perhaps one of the most popular and influential medical books of the time. The literary quality of the work caused Rockefeller's friend, along with tens of thousands of readers, including medical students, doctors and, surprisingly, many laymen to fall under the almost complete "therapeutic nihilism" of a man of the scientific and moral stature of Osler. The book led him to a very clear conclusion: scientific medicine had evolved positively in the second half of the nineteenth century but that development bore no relation to the prevalent therapeutic helplessness. In this sense, Osler's treatise opened many people's eyes to the necessity (and also the opportunity arising from the existing challenge) to strengthen medical education and research. It is clearly evident that this injection of funds and the interest of these new foundations in supporting medical research, produced and continues to produce the favourable consequences familiar to us all and which, eventually, brought about the aforementioned era of "medical miracles" in the last post-war era. All of this eventually translated into an increase in public interest in everything related to health and consequently its eventual adoption by politicians who became convinced of the virtues of supporting medical institutions, establishing those that were needed, and finding the most effective mechanisms to support economically everything related to the sector.

Currently this tendency persists in public health matters thanks to the interest of Bill Gates (1955–) and his Foundation.§

§ Alfred Kopf, MD: This Paradox seems to weigh in on the philanthropic side. However, compared to the support received from foundations, the support from the Public Sector far outweighs them all.

60th Paradox

Western medicine vs. Eastern medicine (Chinese, Hindu, Islamic)

Western medicine does not in fact have any rivals of note. As the effectiveness of its methods have been proven – the use of antibiotics in a wide range of infectious and contagious illnesses for example – it is accepted all over the world with little discussion, contributing to the establishment of an unreserved predominance of Western science and technology. Albeit with some hesitation, ancient Eastern cultures, above all Chinese, Japanese, Korean, Hindu and Islamic cultures, have had to accept this superiority whilst trying to maintain their traditions and customs; a rather uncomfortable situation given the clear implications for many parts of their culture. In the particular case of medicine, a skilful combination of Western technology with the traditional medicine of each country is always sought when possible.

61st Paradox
Scientific medical literature vs. Popular medical literature

Medical knowledge is imparted to medical professionals through scientific books and journals. Before the invention of printing with movable type by Johannes Gutenberg* in around 1450, books in the form of papyrus, parchment, fired clay tablets, etc., were few, costly (they had to be copied by hand), and access to them was limited to just a few educated and interested people. All of this changed radically in the mid-fifteenth century with the advent of the printer. The classic books were translated from Greek to Arabic and Latin, and later to the vernacular languages.

First, the school of medicine in Salerno, and later those of the universities of Padua, Bologna, Paris and Montpellier, were celebrated for their contributions to medicine. They kept interest in the study of the classics alive whilst at the same time creating the essential conditions for the advance and progress of medicine.

The texts of Hippocrates and Galen were closely read and studied by those concerned.

There were authors of great medical works, as in the case of the Persian Ibn Sina, known in the Western world as Avicenna, who produced authentic compilations of medical knowledge of the time.

The most influential medical book of the late 19th/early 20th century is undoubtedly *The Principles and Practice of Medicine*, with the subtitle: *Designed for the use of practitioners and students of medicine*, written by Sir William Osler (1849–1919). Although, as its title suggests, the book was intended for doctors and students of medicine, curiously, and due particularly to its literary qualities (very rare in a medical text

---

* Johannes Gutenberg (*c.*1395–1468), German engraver jeweller and printer

book), it attracted the attention of many laymen. Amongst them was the influential Reverend Frederick T. Gates (1853–1929), a Baptist Minister who as well as working with him on his philanthropic activities was a friend and confidant of the American multimillionaire John D. Rockefeller. In July of 1897 after reading the whole book cover to cover he stated: "I read the whole book without skipping any of it. I speak of this not to commemorate my industry but to celebrate Osler's charm. Osler's Principles and Practice of Medicine is one of the very few scientific books that I have ever read possessed of literary charm. . . . I saw clearly from the work of this able and honest man, that medicine had, with few exceptions, no cures, and that about all that medicine up to 1897 could do was to nurse the patients and alleviate in some degree the suffering. Beyond this, medicine as a science had not progressed.

"It became clear to me that medicine could hardly hope to become a science until medicine should be endowed and qualified men could give themselves to uninterrupted study and investigation, on ample salary, entirely independent of practice." (Rockefeller cited in Corner, 1964: 578–9)

With characteristic North American efficiency and determination, Reverend Gates's fascination with the honesty and literary style of Osler determined a chain of events that eventually led to the creation of the Rockefeller Institute in 1901 and the Rockefeller Foundation in 1913. There followed substantial donations of the same origin to the Faculty of Medicine of the University of Harvard in Boston, and the University of Johns Hopkins and its hospital in Baltimore; these brought about necessary changes in the teaching and practice of medicine with well-known consequences at national and worldwide levels.

Apparently Osler was highly doubtful and reluctant to accept the New York publishing house Appleton's proposition to write the book, for in his opinion it would require a considerable intellectual effort that would temporarily keep him apart from his patients, as in effect it did. Nobody ever imagined that Osler's "therapeutic nihilism", which even came to be described humorously as "paranoia antitherapeuticum baltimorensis" (Hogan, 1999), would come to attract the philanthropic and humanistic attention of one of the richest men in the world and lead to the focus of his munificence in that direction.

The most serious aspect is that Osler was completely right, for although he included the effective therapy of medicines such as iron for anaemia, quinine for malaria, nitroglycerin and amyl nitrite for angina and morphine for pain (which he called GOH–God's Own Medicine), he flatly refused to make space in his book for many of the polypharmaceutical or homeopathic prescriptions that were in vogue at the time.

One edition followed another. By 1905, 105,000 copies had been printed and the royalties reached 54,512 dollars (equivalent to more than a million dollars today), thereby giving the author a relatively, and fairly uncommon, economic independence. By 1947, 500,000 copies of the book in 16 successive editions had been sold, 55 years after the first edition and many years after the death of the author. The book was translated into French, German, Chinese, Spanish and Portuguese.

A century later, with everything that has happened in the field of medical science since then (in partial consequence of the impact produced by the publication of this work), the book would have to be re-written from the first to the last page in order for it to be of any use to doctors and students. In truth the publication of a medical book is a fleeting effort, given that when it is published it is already obsolete and will require multiple revisions.§ For reasons already discussed, the case

§ *Alfred Kopf, MD: The future will no longer be printed Books and Journals but availability via electronic media.*

of Osler's book is notable; its determining influence was due to the enormous prestige of the author and the precision, clarity and amenity of the work.This was summarised by the librarian of the University of Oxford's Bodleian Library, Falconer Madan (1851–1935), when he stated that Osler "had succeeded in making a scientific treatise literature", something which only happens exceptionally. (Cushing, 1940)

There is currently an immense proliferation of scientific and medical journals. It will suffice to mention the few that stand out for their enormous influence.

Amongst the general scientific ones are *Nature* (Great Britain) and *Science* (United States).

Amongst the general medical ones are *The Lancet* (Great Britain), *The Journal of The American Medical Association* or *JAMA* (United States), *The British Medical Journal* (Great Britain), *The New England Journal of Medicine* (United States), *Journal of the Royal Society of Medicine* (Great Britain), *The American Journal of Medicine* (United States) and *Annals of Internal Medicine* (United States).

They are expensive journals, but fortunately summaries of the published articles can be accessed online, and in some cases (for example *The British Medical Journal*) the entire works are available for free, to those people from poorer countries (via the HINARI Programme which was launched in January 2002).

The predominance of English as the *lingua franca* of science and medicine has only emerged in recent decades and the increasingly international authorship of published works in the aforementioned journals is clear indication of the worldwide circulation of these famous publications.

In Venezuela, the most influential scientific journal is *Acta Científica*, whilst the most influential medical journal is *Gaceta Médica de Caracas*. This last one is the official publication of the Academia Nacional de

Medicina; founded by Dr Luis Razetti in 1897, it is the oldest and most prestigious of Venezuela's scientific and medical publications.

As for the general spread of science amongst the uninitiated, that is to say, amongst those members of the public interested in scientific progress but without specific training in the field, *Scientific American* (monthly, United States) and *New Scientist* (weekly, Great Britain) stand out. Once again, English is the international language of communication in this sector.

Public interest in health sciences and medical progress is reflected in the huge number of articles and reports on medicine in the weekly publications of highest international circulation (for example, *Time* and *Newsweek* in the United States and *The Economist* in Great Britain), as well as in the daily press of the most important metropolises of the world, such as New York, London and Paris. Regular columns about medical matters written by distinguished doctors are a characteristic of many of these newspapers.

62nd Paradox
The dissemination of medical knowledge: English vs. Other languages

As established in Paradox 60, as a result of the importance of the United States as a first world power, which is linked to the cultural legacy of the geographic vastness of the dissolved British Empire, the penetration of English on an international level has only increased in the last few decades. This becomes even more evident where science and especially medicine is concerned.

The existing transport and communication facilities made possible by the penetrating and continually growing phenomenon of globalisation naturally contribute to all of this.

Without there existing a definitive strategy for English to be imposed as the *lingua franca* (the equivalent of Latin in the Roman Empire first of all and then throughout the Middle Ages in the universities of Europe), for eminently practical reasons English has gradually become the international language accepted by all. Its rich vocabulary and simple grammar have facilitated its adoption, as much as its phonetic complexities have complicated it. Chinese appears to be its only serious competitor; however, the fact that Chinese is constituted of one language (Mandarin) along with various dialects unintelligible amongst themselves, that it is written using a complicated ideogram system, and that its use is concentrated in China, prevents Chinese from replacing English in the foreseeable future.

On an anecdotal note, I recall that at the World Congress of Dermatology in Berlin in 1987, many German colleagues chose English for their presentations (even though German was one of the four official languages of the meeting), alleging difficulties and inefficiencies of simultaneous translation in such a specialised field. In 2002, at a subsequent congress in Paris not a word was spoken that wasn't English at any of the opening and closing ceremonies. (Even the French have accepted this reality of the contemporary world and have abandoned any attempt to the contrary.)

This does not mean that we will end up speaking only English, but that for practical reasons, if we want our works and writings to be heard and read on an international level, we have to speak and write in English.[§]

Curiously, as the influence of English has become universal, the interest in learning other languages has simultaneously increased in people who speak it as their mother tongue (especially in the United States). Thus we see that the current percentage of bilingual people in the United States reaches 43% in 18 to 29 year olds, drops to 25% in 30 to 49 year olds, and continues diminishing with age. This clearly reveals the interest of the young to learn other languages (with Spanish in first place).

§ *Alfred Kopf, MD: I conclude that a major reason that English has become the "lingua franca" not only in medicine, but also in the world, is its prominence on the Internet.*

63rd Paradox
Science fiction vs. Medical fiction

The growing general public interest in the progress of science, above all in speculation as to what could happen in the future, has given way to the birth and subsequent exponential growth of that literary genre called "science fiction", with an important component that could be called "medical fiction".

The most famous of the authors who have cultivated this literary genre is undoubtedly Jules Verne (1828–1905). In the twentieth century it was Englishmen like George Orwell (pseudonym of Eric Arthur Blair, 1903–1950) and Aldous Huxley (1894–1963) who were most influential, with their perceptive projections for what a twisted exploitation of the scientific and technological potential of the near future could mean for society. Although futurology is essentially an imaginative activity of mere speculation, when it is practised by trained and creative minds it produces novels like those mentioned here whose influence on a whole generation is a singular force.

In Orwell's book *Nineteen Eighty-Four* (published in 1949), and Huxley's *Brave New World* (published in 1932), the action is concentrated on two new technologies, the penetrative influence of which we are now feeling. Orwell's plot focuses on what is today called information technology, and the potential power it offers the State, or "Big Brother", which drives and manipulates the social lives of its citizens via the "Ministry of Truth" and the "Ministry of Love"; it offers an obscurantist vision of what the system of an autocratic and totalitarian government could come to be via the use of these resources.

For his part, Huxley exploits the idea of what the likely progress of biotechnology can achieve, from the in vitro creation of children, to the use of pharmaceuticals and hormones to manipulate the behaviour of people.

Fortunately, as Francis Fukuyama* establishes, more than 50 years after the appearance of these seminal books we can confidently declare that the technological predictions have turned out to be true, but that those of a political nature (like in *Nineteen Eighty-Four*) have turned out to be completely mistaken. The personal computer linked to the Internet is the equivalent of Orwell's "telescreen", "but instead of becoming an instrument of centralisation and tyranny, it led to just the opposite: the democratization of access to information and the decentralization of politics." (Fukuyama, 2006: 307)

Instead of "Big Brother" watching us, people can use the Internet to watch "Big Brother", for which reason governments have been pressurised to publish more information about their activities.

---

* Francis Fukuyama (1952–), American political scientist of Japanese origin

64th Paradox
Freud's psychoanalysis vs. Neuropharmacy

Psychiatry is one of the fields of medicine in which the most dramatic changes of the second half of the twentieth century have been observed, and one of its greatest heroes is undoubtedly Sigmund Freud.* Suffice it to look at the hierarchy established by Michael H. Hart in his work *The 100* in order to understand that Freud has suffered the foreseeable consequences of going from being, as the founder of psycho-analysis, one of the most admired thinkers and discoverer of deep truths about human desires and motivations, to a person who in the view of the current medical profession is only worthy of a footnote at the bottom of a page.

This wide swing of the pendulum of recognition is due in large part to progress in cognitive neuroscience and the development of neuropharmacy.

Four decades ago the wise North American, R. Buckminster Fuller (1895–1983), to whom we can perhaps apply the term of genius given his numerous original contributions to very different fields, drew my attention to the weak service that Freud had paid to medicine. Thanks to his talent, capacity to convince, and express his thoughts in print, he diverted the attention of scholars of mental illnesses towards a methodology without suitable scientific basis, and therefore towards an irretrievable dead end. A similar opinion is attributed to Francis Crick (co-discoverer of the DNA structure) when he states: "By modern standards, Freud can hardly be regarded as a scientist but rather as a physician who had many novel ideas and who wrote persuasively and unusually well. He became the main founder of the new cult of psycho-analysis." (Crick, 1994: 14)

* Sigmund Freud (1856–1939), Austrian doctor – co-founder of psychoanalysis

168

Be that as it may, Freudian thought was built on the premise that mental illnesses (including depression and schizophrenia) were of a primordially psychological nature, resulting from mental dysfunction of the brain.

Such a hypothesis was rather distorted by the chance (perhaps serendipitous) discovery of lithium for manic-depressive illnesses by the Australian psychiatrist John Cade (1912–80) in 1948.

Then came a new generation of psycho-pharmaceuticals with Prozac and Ritalin at the forefront, in what has been called "the Neurotransmitter Revolution" (Masters & McGuire, 1994), and with it the possibility of effectively treating those suffering from such afflictions.

This type of pharmaceutical blocks the reabsorption of serotonin at the level of the nerve synapse, thereby increasing the level of serotonin in the brain.

It is stated that currently Prozac (and drugs like Zoloft and Paxil) have been used to treat 28 million North Americans.

For its part, Ritalin (methylphenidate), a stimulant drug related to methamphetamine, is widely used to treat Attention Deficit Hyperactivity Disorder (ADHD), a hyperactivity problem commonly associated with boys incapable of sitting quietly at their desks in class.

Fukuyuma has drawn attention to what he qualifies as "disconcerting symmetry" between Prozac and Ritalin. Where on the one hand the first pharmaceutical is prescribed to depressed women who suffer from a lack of self-esteem, on the other hand, the second is given to boys who are restless in class. According to this interpretation, the two sexes are being trapped in what he calls "androgynous median personality", or "self-satisfied and socially compliant", which is "politically correct" in contemporary North American society. (Fukuyuma, 2002: 52)

If we look at it this way, it's evident that a single author interested in manipulating human behaviour, or "Big Brother", doesn't really exist, rather it is governments, teachers, parents, doctors and others who have the ability to intervene in this type of "social control".

The public seeks pills not only to control feminine fertility, but also to increase intelligence, memory, emotional sensitivity, sex, and even to reduce aggression and violence.

65th Paradox
The criminalisation of certain drugs vs. General use of the same or similar drugs

There is undoubted ambivalence in behaviour towards psychotropic medicine and drugs with very similar pharmacological properties to methylenedioxymethamphetamine (MDMA), known in popular North American slang as "Ecstasy", a stimulant that is chemically very similar to methamphetamine and widely and illegally used in nightclubs and other places of night-time fun.

Our mixed feelings towards drugs that have a "feel good" effect on the people who consume them, but no obvious therapeutic indications, are clear.

Whilst on the one hand, pharmaceuticals like Prozac and Ritalin are prescribed to millions of patients, "Ecstasy", marijuana and cocaine, drugs which so far do not have clear therapeutic indications, are criminalised. What possible scientific or moral basis can there be for the declaration of marijuana as illegal, when the use and abuse of nicotine and alcohol are permitted?

However, it is possible that attitudes may change in the future, as with the case of marijuana which is said to induce a certain level of well-being in terminally ill cancer patients (where there is no risk of future addiction).§ This has been the general approach of the medical profession in relation to the use of morphine in terminal patients with different types of pain.

§ *Alfred Kopf, MD: A number of States in the USA have passed laws approving the establishment of marijuana growing farms to sell the product for "medicinal use" (e.g. epilepsy, especially in children).*

66th Paradox
Prolongation of life vs. Quality of life

The foreseeable medium term consequences of the age projections currently available are truly alarming for the developed countries of the North. Although until now the principal cause for concern has derived from a giant growing mass of retirees and pensioners alongside a clearly decreasing group of people who work and produce, the consequences of the prolongation of life, contemporary medicine's great achievement, are many and varied, with the majority being negative for the strong and healthy society to which we all aspire.

The paradigm of the medical profession establishes, without doubt, that every action intended to defeat disease and prolong life is positive.

Until a generation ago we were not in a position to judge the trap that we had fallen into, a potentially "Faustian contract" where in order to obtain the supposed benefits of long life we have seriously compromised the "quality" of that life by permitting people to pass their eightieth and ninetieth years, which as we are well aware does not occur without punishment.

One of the gravest problems we are facing is that of the dependence and general disability of the old. In a society where family tends to disperse, and where the responsibilities of the adult generation that works and produces is centred, with some reason, on their young and adolescent children, a sense of responsibility for their parents and the older generation is gradually fading to the point where it has almost disappeared.

The most serious threat that hangs over old people is Alzheimer's disease, which causes brain damage and leads to loss of memory and dementia. At 65 years of age, only one in a hundred will develop this illness; at 85 years it's one in six.

Two categories have been classified in this advanced period of life. Category I extends from the age of retirement to 80 years of age. Although currently variable, it is understood from the Bismarck era, when social security was introduced in Germany, that the age of retirement is 65 years old. At that time, the end of the nineteenth century, very few actually reached this age. Category I is possibly the age at which citizens of developed countries hope to enjoy a deserved rest, travel, and spend time on their "hobbies" (good health permitting).

Category II is much more problematic. Extending beyond 80 years, it is during this period that a growing dependency is observed, where sensorial, locomotive and mental capacities continually decline before reaching the degrading situation of infantile dependency.

Stem cell research could resolve the problem of creating new organs to replace those already spent and exhausted in their functional capacity, but if these promises don't coincide with an effective treatment for the evil of Alzheimer's, what purpose is served by thousands of old people who live up to the age of 120 but are confined for many years, even decades, to old people's homes? 122.45 years is the human lifespan record, established by the French supercentenarian Madame Jeanne Calment (1875–1997), who lived her whole life in Arles in the South of France.

Every species has a well-established upper age limit. Will our species' maximum age have increased in recent years? The answer to this question appears to be affirmative as it is reported that from 1969 to 1999 the maximum length of life increased by 1.1 years per decade (www.therubins.com/aging/maximum.htm).

I recall the case of a distinguished intellectual and politician from Colombia, who at a very young age had married a very intelligent and qualified woman who was some years older than him. He described his very special relationship with her by saying that he and his wife had experienced the whole range of possibilities of this type of relationship. At the beginning she was his guide, inspiration and teacher, then she was his companion for many years, and at the end of his life he came to be her nurse, such was the level of dependency of the old lady.

When towards the end of his long life Arturo Uslar Pietri* was asked how he was, he replied, "old age is a shipwreck". What better metaphor to describe the tragedy represented by old age!

Indeed, the moment arrives at the end of the biological cycle in which death appears a blessing if the only way one can stay alive is as a vegetable.

A colleague was once asked by a patient for advice on living a long life, he answered: "If you want to live for many years, choose your grandparents well", indicating the importance of genes and inheritance in determining the hazardous factor of the end of every human being's life. The eternal controversy of nature vs. nurture extends to this field of life expectancy, for as long as the "genetic lottery" provides the "winning card" that offers the possibility of a long life, man has in his hands the ability to prolong his existence through a healthy lifestyle, avoiding excesses, eating healthily, exercising, abstaining from smoking and excessive alcohol consumption, etc. Given the problems of longevity after a certain advanced age and while the therapeutic weapons against Alzheimer's Disease and senile dementia are not yet in our reach, perhaps a long life might not be so exceedingly desirable.

* Arturo Uslar Pietri, Venezuelan politician and intellectual

174

67th Paradox
Lifestyle diseases vs. Environmental diseases

These two types of disease are intimately connected to each other in the sense that lifestyle represents a change in the environment.

Aside from those illnesses caused by the medical act (iatrogenic illnesses), a vast variety of illnesses, such as obesity, are caused by life-style, whereas others may be derived from the environment in which we are immersed, for example, occupational illnesses.

It is said that lifestyle diseases, also known as diseases of civilisation, "are a group of illnesses that occur more frequently in industrialised countries and whose risk of contraction depends in part on the prevailing conditions of life and life expectancy (diseases of longevity)". (*Wikipedia*, 26 October 2014)

This concept was born in France in the mid-nineteenth century when the doctor Stanislas Tanchou (1791–1850) noticed a difference between the incidences of diseases like cancer or insanity in urban and rural environments.

Industrialisation and the introduction of numerous synthetic products add new diseases to the immense repository of occupational illnesses every day.

Who would have imagined the risks to which students and teachers would be exposed when rural schools were designed and built with cheap insulated roofs containing asbestos? The possibility of developing asbestosis and its potential consequences (malignant mesothelioma) were unknown at the time.

How many similar experiences await us in the future? Every new substance that is introduced to the market carries a potential risk, and it is practically impossible to determine with any accuracy the dormant damaging effects that may arise in the medium and long term; hence the new fashion, which is currently so in vogue, of using only "organic" products which are supposedly free of the contamination imposed by man in his desire to improve his economic yield.§

§ *Alfred Kopf, MD: It is fitting to mention here the man-made reduction (by release of atomic halogens into the stratosphere) of stratospheric and tropospheric ozone (a natural "sunscreen"), leading to the ever-increasing incidence of cancers of the skin, including malignant melanoma.*

68th Paradox
Curative medicine vs. Preventative medicine

These are not actually opposing or contradictory actions, in fact they are complementary. The ideal would be prevention instead of cure, for every time that prevention is possible, and with it the avoidance of illness, we can be certain that there will be a considerable saving in the human suffering and costs that run in parallel in these types of situation.

These days when the traditional enemies of infectious disease and malnutrition have been overcome by modern medicine, the principal causes of incapacity and premature death are attributed to old age and behavioural factors. It is estimated that by 2020 tobacco use will be the biggest cause of preventable illness in the world.

Modern means of communication, such as the Internet with its health sites, blogs and social networks, offer extraordinary opportunities to educate the greater public on the prevention of numerous illnesses. In fact this is happening without the existence of a functional coordination to achieve it. Cell phones, especially smart phones, singularly lend themselves to preventative campaigns via short educational messages (such as a "tweet") that target risk groups by age, sex, place of residence, etc. Taking into account the level of penetration of the cell phone in Venezuela, it is easy to understand the potential of this medium; in order for this potential to be reached the health authorities, specialised medicine communities, insurance companies and mobile phone companies would need to come to an agreement.

69th Paradox
Medical illustrations vs. Pictorial art

Should medical illustrations be viewed as an art form? According to the art history guru Ernst Gombrich,* medical illustration is an art form that is both representational and conceptual.

The Renaissance genius Leonardo da Vinci (1492–1519) introduced shadow technique to give a tri-dimensional effect and established the techniques and conventions of anatomical art that are essential to medical illustration.

Andreas Vesalius (1514–64) was born in Brussels and trained as a doctor at the universities of Leuven, Paris, Brussels and Padua. It was in Padua where he obtained his doctorate at 23 years of age and where, on the following day, he was named Professor of Anatomy and Surgery. In 1543 he published his famous book *De humani corporis fabrica libri septem*, of which Sir William Osler claimed ". . . it is the greatest book ever printed, from which modern medicine dates". (Clinical Anatomy Associates, 2015) It consists of 200 anatomical drawings; the carved blocks of wood for the illustrations were executed in Venice, probably by artists recruited from Titian's workshops, under the direct supervision of Vesalius and with the printing done in Basel. The art of medical illustration has had distinguished representation in every generation since the publication of his book.

Before the development of colour photography to its current level, there was a need to visually depict skin diseases. It's therefore worth remembering the famous wax "moulages", or sculptures, of Jules Baretta (1833–1923) who sculpted more than 2,000 for the museum of

* Ernst Gombrich (1909–2001), art historian born in Austria and a naturalised British citizen

the hospital of Saint-Louis in Paris. These permitted the teaching of dermatology to medical students and future dermatologists, and are still displayed as works of art at the same hospital, which, having been very well maintained since its inauguration by King Henry IV in 1607, is considered an architectural gem in the "City of Light" (*La Ville Lumière*).

It's appropriate to pay tribute here to the extraordinary coloured chalk anatomical drawings of the great anatomy maestro of several generations of Venezuelan doctors, Dr José Izquierdo. I recall seeing his Chinese ink drawing of what was supposedly the skull of the Liberator Simón Bolívar, which he discovered in the Bolívar family crypt in Caracas Cathedral and which caused a well-known controversy.

70th Paradox
Damage limitation vs. Damage elimination

There is a modern movement that is headed in the direction of "damage limitation", especially in the context of drug abuse, which has such a detrimental effect on health.

Instead of defining drug consumption as an illness or a concession of moral character, this new position applies an approach that is both human and practical. It is an attempt to help addicts to understand the risks they are running and thereby make their own decisions and fix their own objectives.

The research gathered by the Jellinek Institute in the Netherlands, named in honour of E. M. Jellinek,* is carefully analysed in the book edited by G. Alan Marlatt.† It offers much to ponder upon; its criticism of the recent strategy of "zero tolerance" in the war against drugs, led him to claim that "zero tolerance + zero compassion = zero".

* E. M. Jellinek (1890–1963), American biostatistician, physiologist and alcoholism expert
† G. Alan Marlatt (1941–2011), American psychologist and alcoholism scholar

71st Paradox
Natural pharmaceutical products vs. Synthetic pharmaceuticals

Recent history has taught us how both of these approaches are widely used by the industry in order to supply a market that is ever hungry for new medicines against diseases for which we previously lacked demonstrably effective weapons, or for more effective pharmaceuticals than those currently in use.

There is no doubt that medicine has much to gain from the great keeper of biodiversity that we call nature. In general, after a potential pharmaceutical is identified in nature and its medicinal action has been proven, it is then produced synthetically, often at a lower cost.

The pharmaceutical products currently in use are largely derived from wild species. In the United States close to a quarter of medical prescriptions are for substances of a plant extraction. Another 13% come from micro-organisms and 3% from animals. It is incredible but true that nine out of every ten pharmaceuticals are derived from organisms. In 1980, the sale of these drugs without prescription (on free sale to the public in the US) was estimated to total some 20 billion dollars and 84 billion worldwide.

Despite its obvious potential, only a tiny fraction of biodiversity has been used for medicine. The narrowness of this base is illustrated by the predominance of Ascomycota mushrooms in the control of bacterial diseases. Although only 30,000 species of Ascomycota mushrooms have been studied – and there are over 64,000 species in total – they have already provided 85% of the antibiotics currently in use.

Bio-exploration is the study of biodiversity in the search for potentially useful natural resources. Those countries with a significant proportion of tropical rain forest in their territory, such as Venezuela (with the majority in the Orinoco basin and part of the Amazon and

Essequibo basins), have exceptional potential wealth as well as an unavoidable responsibility to conserve the forest and with it the eco-systems that host a number of fauna and flora species whose therapeutic possibilities remain almost completely unexplored by scientific research.

Experience has taught us that due to the thin topsoil in that part of the world, felling trees for timber and giving the earth over to livestock and agriculture, provides no sustainable output, but just a handful of harvests (in contrast with the sustained farming of land generations ago in temperate climates). For this reason, these practices, although tempting in the present, have a very limited economic and social future.

This is why many non-governmental organisations (NGOs) are so enthusiastically dedicated to convincing the governments of those countries that still possess sizeable amounts of tropical forest that there exist alternatives. These alternatives, an intelligent combination of eco-tourism, bio-exploration, and perhaps in the near future the exchange of virgin land for carbon credits – one of the strategies promoted by the conservationists to diminish global warming – may turn out to be more profitable than felling trees and the fleetingly successful agricul-ture that may occur on the land.

According to figures by the Food and Agriculture Organisation of the United Nations (FAO), Venezuela still has 457,000 km^2 of tropical forest, which is nearly half of its territory. However, with deforestation at a rate of 5,990 km^2 per year (1980–1990), which translates as 1.31% per year, which is higher than Bolivia (1.16%), Brazil (0.9%), Colombia (0.68%) and Peru (0.4%), and lower only than Ecuador (1.98%) out of all of the Amazonian countries, the future doesn't look bright. Venezuela again finds itself in an unfavourably critical situation, even compared with other countries in the region, which are all besieged by the same temptations and short-sightedness in their public conservation policies.

It's appropriate to mention here that in its temperate zone Venezuela must be mindful of the past: as previously explained reversing the use of land for a large part of its territory is not an option. More than 60% of forests in temperate zones have been lost to deforestation to provide land for agriculture (as well as 45% of tropical rain forest and 70% of tropical dry forest).

The good news in all of this negative reality is that NGOs have become more creative and have created programmes to obtain donations to buy the commercial debt of countries at a significant discount (this often concerns developing countries that are fiercely in debt, with some facing bankruptcy). They then dedicate these funds to buying land and converting it into reserves, to environmental education and to improving the management of those reserves that already exist. Countries like Bolivia, Costa Rica, the Dominican Republic, Ecuador, Mexico, Madagascar, Zambia, the Philippines and Poland have favoured the implementation of this type of strategy.

Unfortunately, it is clear that Venezuela is once again trailing behind in developing conservationist strategies like those outlined here.

Dr Rice is an economist, ecologist, and the architect of a conservation concessions programme called "warp-speed conservation", which is undertaken by Conservation International for whom he works. With the possibility of being able to check the progress of the programme and its successful implementation in Venezuela's neighbouring country Guyana, I visited Dr Rice at his offices in Washington D.C. in May 2002 in order to find out more details about his programme, which was included in *Scientific American* in May 2002.

Based on the success of this type of programme, which is born of a realistic view of the issue at hand, current owners of tropical forest (usually either governments or private owners) will be able to decide if their economic interests remain favoured under this type of agreement,

183

and moreover serve the conservation cause, which is of paramount importance to the future of our species.

Three decades ago the *Consejo Nacional para Investigaciones Científicas y Tecnológicas* (National Council for Scientific and Technological Research or CONICIT) in Costa Rica was introduced to the work of the biochemist and ethnobotanist Dr Conrad Gorinsky (1936–). The son of a Polish immigrant and a descendant of Cacique Indians from the Rupununi area of Guyana, Gorinsky was educated in the UK. It was through the then Venezuelan Ambassador to Great Britain, Dr Juan Manuel Sucre Trías (1940–83), that Grinsky's work on the development of the new discipline, ethnobotany, in which he was particularly competent, was recommended to CONICIT. Ethnobotany is based on the oral tradition of Amerindians, where the medical properties of certain plants are passed from generation to generation. A visit was arranged to establish a cooperative programme of research in this new and interesting area for Venezuela, but it was abruptly dropped without the invitee being informed of the reasons for it ending that way. All of this leads one to suspect that Venezuela has a complex about sitting down and negotiating, and a lack of understanding of the fact that an intelligently managed negotiation table brings advantageous agreements for both parties. Perhaps our lack of experience and past negative transactions, coupled with being sustained by the oil wealth that transformed us into a rentier country lacking in creativity and initiatives, has created a negative psychology that paralyses creative action.

72nd Paradox
Knowledge gathered from medicine vs. Knowledge from the basic sciences that feed it

"That which is a day older than you is a day wiser."

Although the scientific component of medicine is derived from the knowledge and innovations of scientific research in basic sciences (especially biochemistry, biophysics, molecular biology, immunology and genetics) and has provided doctors with some formidable tools and added an infallible prestige to their therapeutic strategies, we should not be deceived. For as Sir Peter Medawar* says, scientific research is in essence "the art of the soluble", that is to say the art of what can be resolved (1968). It is therefore easy to imagine that the "insolubles" (those which are not resolved) constitute, if not the majority of problems, then at least those of greater depth and reach, including the origin of life, the afterlife, the meaning of human existence, and many others that form the substance of philosophy and religion.

The fact that medicine has a great advantage over the other sciences in being older and driven since the time of Hippocrates by a definitive common aim, means there is less temptation for it to fall into the contagious dogma of the almighty power of science, which has gradually permeated contemporary society and momentarily blinded its capacity to comprehend the true limitations of its action.

* Sir Peter Medawar (1915–87), British biologist, recipient of the Nobel Prize for Medicine, 1960

73rd Paradox
Synthesis vs. Analysis in medical thought

Philosophically speaking, this paradox covers all realms of human thought, however, at a reductive level it boils down to general medical thinking (in which the family doctor and the internist are currently more rigorously and intellectually trained, compared with specialists who have an even more reduced vision).

On the meaning of synthesis and analysis, I have been tempted to reproduce a personal anecdote from *Venezuela Analítica*, which is relevant to the subject:

Nearly four decades ago I had the privilege of meeting and addressing Mr Buckminster Fuller (1895–1983) when he visited Caracas to see an exhibition put on by the United States Embassy in the *Zona Rental* of the *Ciudad Universitaria*. He was clearly an exceptional man (he could qualify as my "unforgettable celebrity"), a true genius, in that his mind was of the highest level to which man's intellectual faculties can reach (and I am very economical with this level of praise for people I have met). A true renaissance man, he had mastered a great variety of scientific and humanistic disciplines, and offered to each of them truly valuable and original contributions. It is difficult to know with any level of accuracy in which discipline he was most outstanding; he has been called an architect, cartographer, geometrician, futurist, teacher and poet interchangeably. The *Encyclopaedia Britannica* describes him as "one of the most original thinkers of the second half of the twentieth century" (*Encyclopaedia Britannica Online*, 24 August 2015). Fuller had been invited to Venezuela to inaugurate the exhibition where he was displaying one of his famous geodesic domes – the only great dome that can rest directly on the floor as a complete structure and the only type of construction with no theoretical limits to its possible dimensions.

One fine day during his stay in Caracas, Mr Fuller surprised me with the well-known question: which is man's most important invention? And before I had finished mentally running through the habitual long list, he answered me emphatically: the computer. And this, one has to remember, was at the beginning of the 1970s. His restless mind was already practising daring futurology and imagining with complete accuracy what would happen in the next 40 years.

It is easy to imagine my curiosity to understand the reasons for which a man of his intellectual capacity would have this opinion on such a complex and contested subject. He told me that the days of the human species, like all other biological species, were numbered, and that the high degree of specialisation that had developed would condition our species' extinction. But suddenly, with the invention of the computer, man had managed to "buy time" for survival on the planet, for the wonderful computer is more trustworthy than a human brain in one of two principal tasks: analysis. Thus man, liberated from these complex and tedious functions, is able to concentrate on the most sublime of functions, that of synthesis.

Ever since then I have had great respect for the computer, and nothing that has happened in the last 40 years has surprised me, in fact it has only served to verify and prove Buckminster Fuller's hypothesis.

For this reason I wholly endorse any initiative intended to train our population in the use of computers and particularly in suitable instruments to gain access to information via the Internet.

For the first time in history, developing countries (a euphemism for under-developed) can reduce that immense breach between the informed and uninformed (or ignorant) and, if they choose their priorities well, make real and permanent progress in improving their quality of life. Current technology is offering us a true revolution that we must not miss.

The importance of libraries and their immense cost until some years ago compared with the recent development of "online search engines" (like Google) are a prime example of the Internet's contribution and how it has "democratised access to information". For years I thought that the lack of well-endowed and functional libraries was one of the greatest cultural barriers to the development of poorer nations, and suddenly thanks to information technology, that previously insurmountable obstacle has been dispelled before our eyes.

Another phenomenon worthy of mention is the appearance and current influence of *Wikipedia*, a digital encyclopaedia that is free to use. It grows on a daily basis, in multiple languages, and has the capacity for almost instantaneous correction; it is a new and incredibly valuable instrument for the cultural universe.

74th Paradox
Rural (and tropical) medicine vs. District community medicine

Until only a generation ago the Venezuelan population was mainly rural and therefore exposed to the generally infectious and parasitic tropical diseases that are prevalent in the hot climates of the world (between the Tropic of Cancer at 23° 26' 16" north of the Equator and the Tropic of Capricorn with the same coordinates to the South).

With the growing urbanisation of the country (a common phenomenon in developing nations but especially pronounced in Venezuela where 90% of the population now live in cities), the issue of rural medical care has become, at least partially, that of district medical care, with the big cities surrounded as they are by shanty towns (or *"ranchos"* – the name given to the shack-like houses that make up these areas). They have sprung up on uninhabited land, such as has occurred in the hills surrounding Caracas, with no planning or services whatsoever. Today their inhabitants represent a significant percentage of the country's population.

It is evident that the practice of "rural medicine" that is asked of recently graduated medicine students in Venezuela must move, at least partially, to outpatient clinics in the districts of big cities, where the population with lower economic resources reside en masse, although the more remote rural areas must not be abandoned. Venezuela, as well as other countries on the road to development, stopped being a rural country years ago and became an urban one instead, with populous cities surrounded by districts of shanty towns or *favelas*.

75th Paradox
New diseases of known aetiology vs. New and little understood aetiologies

A typical case, with current validity, is the disease commonly known as "Mad Cow Disease" and its relationship to Creutzfeldt-Jakob disease in humans.

"Mad Cow Disease, Bovine spongiform encephalopathy, is a disease caused by prions, which can be transmitted to human beings via the consumption of parts of infected animals, above all nervous tissue." (*Wikipedia*, 24 August 2015)

In 1996 a variant of Creutzfeldt-Jakob disease related to the epidemic of spongiform encephalopathy in bovine livestock was identified in humans.

For its part, Creutzfeldt-Jakob disease "is a neurological disorder, with hereditary genetic forms, produced by a protein called prion (PrP). Although hereditary and infectious cases are perfectly documented, the cause of the appearance of prion is unknown in the majority of reported cases. This is an illness of a degenerative nature with a mortal prognosis that affects approximately one person in a million (prevalence of $1:10^6$) on a global scale." (*Wikipedia*, 24 August 2015)

76th Paradox
Diseases of deficiency vs. Diseases of affluence

"If a choice must be made, free school meals are more important for the health of poor children than immunization programmes, and both are more effective than hospital beds." (McKeown, 1979: 120)

Thanks to modern transportation, the famines that caused the death of thousands and millions of people in the past are unlikely to occur in the future. This type of catastrophe, caused by a prolonged period of lack of food in a community, leading to malnutrition and death and potentially the outbreak of infectious diseases, is therefore a phenomenon of the past and consigned to history, at least in the majority of the countries in the world (isolated cases are still recorded in Bangladesh, Ethiopia, Somalia and the countries of Sub-Saharan Africa, which received almost immediate effective international aid). The Great Famine in Ireland in the 1840s stands out in history; caused by the failure of potato crops, it led to a significant migration phenomenon.

The disappearance of this type of disaster is undoubtedly due to improved distribution of food, a consequence of better and faster transport means. It has been firmly established that improved human nutrition, in quantity and quality and including animal proteins, has translated over time into an increase in the physical size and strength of entire populations. During the Gallipoli battles of the First World War, the Turks were surprised to notice the difference in stature between English fighters (who had come from the congested cities of the runaway industrial revolution) and the Australians and New Zealanders (with the same ancestors, but who were well-fed on sheep or cow meat); a case which is often cited.

But whilst it is true that death by starvation is a rare phenomenon these days, for the omnipresent poor of the developing world it is the principal cause of a great number of health problems, which can be grouped under the headings of malnutrition and undernourishment.

Malnutrition is defined as an unbalanced diet due to the predominance of some nutrients and the scarcity of others, meaning that the body's needs are not adequately met.

Particular deficiencies include vitamin deficiency, or hypovitaminosis, as commonly it is the partial, not the complete, absence of vitamins that leads to the development of diseases such as scurvy (Vitamin C deficiency), Osteomalacia (Vitamin D deficiency), Pellagra (Nicotinic Acid deficiency), etc.

An extreme case of malnourishment is Kwashiorkor, a syndrome caused by an intense protein deficiency, principally observed in children of a young age and characterised by oedema, pigment alterations in the skin and hair, hepatic alterations and a distended abdomen. At first glance, oedema can be confused with weight excess, and changes in skin and hair pigmentation, towards a reddish tone, make the person look healthy, which can deceive those who are unaware of the symptoms.

The human metabolic system can endure extreme food deprivation, as was proven on a large scale by the Nazi concentration camps of the Second World War. It is necessary to re-nourish those who suffer from this type of advanced malnutrition little by little. Brothers Joseph and Theodore Gillman, who were doctors and specialists in nutrition in South Africa, predicted the risks of eager and uncontrolled feeding of emaciated prisoners released from concentration camps, and wrote a letter to the leaders of Western democracies, alerting them to the potential danger.

Unfortunately, a lack of caution and control led to many cases of quick death caused by an excess of food, in men, women and children who had been used to eating starvation rations for months or years. It is similar to what occurs when the octane level in gasoline is radically changed in a car.

Malnutrition is sometimes caused by more than economic problems i.e. extreme poverty, it can occur for cultural reasons too.

Deficiencies are more serious in pregnant women and infants, as they can cause severe problems in development with permanent consequences, which is why nutrition programmes for children and their mothers are so important.

At the other extreme, an excess of nutrition intake, caused by wealth or affluence and characterised by an excess of body weight through the accumulation of fatty tissue, is taking place on a large scale in the industrialised countries of the North. This is especially the case in the United States where according to recent statistics obesity affects 61% of the population.

Anthropometrically speaking, obesity is when the body mass index (weight in kilograms/square of the height in metres) exceeds 30 kg/m^2.

Obesity has become one of the gravest public health problems of recent years.

77th Paradox
Environmental diseases vs. Lifestyle diseases

"There is nothing new under the sun", says an old proverb, and the following paragraph confirms it.

"These days we live in a world that is deeply dedicated to material things, just like in the late Roman world. For example, the Romans of the IV Century were obsessed with health, diet and exercise. They spent a greater length of time in baths and health clubs than in churches, temples, libraries or courts of law. They were devoted to the act of consuming. A man's reputation could be built by spending more than his neighbour, even if he had to borrow the money to do it. And, if he couldn't pay his creditors, he was honoured for having made a noble attempt at being somebody . . . They were excited by travel, the news and shows . . . They were fascinated by fame and they didn't care how it was achieved. If you were sufficiently famous, the fact that you might be a thief, or worse, was ignored or pardoned . . . The Romans were principally interested in being successful, and they interpreted this as looking after today and leaving tomorrow to look after itself. They were proud, greedy and vain. In short, they were a lot like us."

The Romans enjoyed a period of civilisation during their *Pax Romana* era, and, demonstrating the similarities highlighted above, this has also been the case for more than half a century in industrialised countries and the powerful classes of developing countries with the *Pax Americana* era. The leisure afforded by the affluence that civilisation brings with it leads to "lifestyle diseases", amongst which being overweight stands out.

A great number of occupational illnesses can be included in the environmental illnesses category, such as silicosis and asbestosis, which are produced by the respective inhalation of particles of silica or asbestos over a prolonged period of time. Until a few years ago non-smokers could fall victim to an environmental illness when they were exposed to cigarette smoke from smokers in public places. Fortunately, today public awareness has led to regulations that are more and more restrictive for smokers, thereby avoiding the possibility of this vice being indiscriminately harmful to third parties.

Lifestyle diseases are those caused by a person's lifestyle, they are predominant in a large number of human beings from developed countries and are characterised by excess of food, lack of physical exercise (and at times, intellectual exercise), and are often accompanied by the consumption of tobacco and excessive consumption of alcohol.

Without a shadow of a doubt, the lifestyle adopted by a large part of the population of affluent countries represents the greatest assault on health. This can be controlled by health education programmes adapted to specific situations, according to the culture and characteristics of each group and nation.

78th Paradox
Solitary old age vs. Old people's homes

With the increasing dissolution of the nuclear family along with the disappearance of domestic service, old people, many of them widows or widowers (as the coordination of a couple's simultaneous death is impossible), spend the last days of their life in solitude or old people's homes; an additional tragedy in the "shipwreck" represented by old age.

From a psychological point of view, solitude is a potential threat that affects every human being, and which becomes more real as we age. Even in those countries with advanced social security, such as Spain, a suitable solution to the problem has not been found. In Madrid, at the time of writing, there are 132,595 people over the age of 64 living in complete solitude, of which some 50,000 are over 80 years old.

The issue is that pronounced old age is in itself an illness, or more accurately, a poly-illness. The senses progressively decrease in their normal keenness, and the so-called "ailments of old age" are actually symptoms and signs of incapacity and insufficiency in the different organs, apparatus and systems that make up the human body. Admittedly, these symptoms do not all occur at the same time or with identical intensity, with no predetermined pattern or consideration of the breakthrough diseases that they can provoke at any moment; each person is different with some failing earlier than others. Such was the supposition of René Descartes* who simplified the ageing process by comparing our anatomy and physiology with a machine, where the breakdown of one part, leads to the entire machine being unable to adequately function. For this reason the problems of old age are medical as well as social, and the solutions, palliative as they necessarily

* René Descartes (1596–1650), French philosopher and mathematician

are, ultimately fall to medical professionals. We are far from discovering the elixir of youth or something similar, in spite of the promises and "enchantments" offered by, amongst others, Swiss clinics with their cell injections and similar procedures with no scientific basis. In the majority of cases, by correcting our lifestyle (ideal weight, exercise, appropriate diet, abstaining from tobacco, moderation of alcohol, etc.) we can aspire to sustain a certain quality of life for a few more years. But after that what we can honestly predict for the beginning of the 21st century seems to fall under the heading of science fiction, or more specifically, medical fiction (a growing genre). Implants can, and in fact do, successfully replace essential components, for example: the opaque crystalline in cataracts; the cochlear implant for hearing; or even a joint (hip, knee or shoulder) for arthrosis. The materials with which these implants and prostheses are made (in the case of substituting parts of the skeleton) are more and more sophisticated and have a life that often exceeds the patient's lifespan. Transplants (especially the kidney, but also the liver, heart, lungs, bone marrow, cornea, bone and even pancreatic islets), skin grafts or organs (skin, fat, fascia, cartilage, bone, etc.), and the promise of what the implantation of stem cells into grossly deficient organs and tissues can come to mean, are partial solutions that can prolong the useful life of a given patient. However, unfortunately, up until now, in the moment in which I write these lines, there exists a general pessimism about similar progress in regards to the functioning of that central organ which is fundamental to a bare minimum of quality of life: the human brain.

As I have already implied, old age in itself is a disease and the fact that there exists a medical specialism for the study and health care of the ageing (geriatrics) proves this.

Contemporary society, especially in industrialised countries, has increased the average lifespan of its population, which admittedly has an upper limit that appears to be quite inflexible. This, along with a decrease in the birth rate, will inevitably bring about a considerable increase in the old-age population.

Old people's homes do not solve the overall emotional problems of the old person. Whilst it is true that they are housed with people of the same generation, they are still strangers to one another. The fact remains that they are isolated and separated from their family, who may visit regularly, or occasionally, when work and other obligations permit. Moreover, it is a costly way of resolving the problem, one that not all family groups can afford.

79th Paradox
Therapeutic friendship vs. Commercialisation and defensive medicine

We understand therapeutic friendship to be the affectionate relationship or friendship that can be established between a doctor and patient, which substantially contributes to the success of the medical act. It produces in the doctor a greater interest, empathy, and even concern, to help the patient find suitable solutions to the health problems that affect them, inspiring in them the necessary confidence to closely follow the prescribed treatment and advice.

This relationship is the fundamental opposite of the commercialisation of medicine, which conceives of medicine as a mere service activity provided in exchange for money. Medical activity cannot and should not be understood as a simple economic activity. It is clear from age-old experience that those who practise medicine with only material gain in mind, end up being indifferent to the real needs of the patient, and sooner or later this can lead to medical malpractice.

Defensive medicine contributes to the commercialisation of medicine. This approach aims to avoid medical malpractice claims and is often achieved via an excessive and unnecessary number of laboratory tests and examinations, even when a reasonably precise diagnosis has already been reached. It clearly causes an unnecessary increase in the cost of the medical act and the loss of the patient's confidence in their treating doctor.

80th Paradox
The wisdom of the body vs. The stupidity of the body

"The Wisdom of the Body" is a book title that has been used by various medical writers. It is a completely justified reflection of their admiration for the precision, within great complexity, with which the regulatory interior mechanisms of the body work.

For example, the body's respiratory rhythm of approximately 16 respirations per minute; or a cardiac rhythm which can fluctuate between 60 and 100 pulsations per minute; or body temperature of 36.5 to 37.5 degrees centigrade (according to whether taken from skin or the oral or rectal mucosa); or systolic blood pressure of between 12 and 14 cm Hg and diastolic pressure between 6 and 8 cm Hg; and so on. There are hundreds of other constant values with minor fluctuations, which permit the maintenance of the body's complex balances and homeostasis (the balance in the composition of the internal average of the body, regulated by the endocrine and nervous systems).

This title was also used by the medical writer and professor of surgery at Yale University, Sherwin B. Nuland (1930–2014) for his informative book on medicine *The Wisdom of the Body*. The same title has also been repeatedly used by notable medical scientists: in 1923 by Ernest Starling (1866–1927) as the title of the prestigious *Harveian Oration* at the Royal College of Physicians in London; in 1932 by Walter B. Cannon (1871–1945), professor of physiology at Harvard, in another seminal book widely known for having coined the term "homeostasis" for the human body's extraordinary self-regulation; and Sir Charles Sherrington (1857–1952) in the twelve Gifford lectures delivered at the University of Edinburgh in 1937 to 1938.

However, this wisdom also has its limitations; these exceptions to the rule were named by the doctor and researcher Marcel Roche

(1920–2003) as "the stupidity of the body". Under this title, a sharp observer like Marcel included the group of so-called "auto-immune disorders", where an abnormal reaction against constituent elements of the body's own tissues leads to pathological processes that affect a person's health.

81st Paradox
Scientific research using stem cells vs. Foetus cells

The hope of being able to use stem cells for the reconstruction of tissues, organs and systems in a human body that is damaged, insufficient or decrepit appears to be a real possibility within the reach of the technology at our disposal.

Incidentally, the Swiss doctor Paul Niehans (1882–1971), who became famous for his rejuvenation treatments (and who is attributed with curing Pope Pius XII of persistent hiccups), laid the foundations for cellular therapy by using sheep cells. His procedure had no scientific basis at all as it used cells from another species, which, when transplanted into a human being, would be identified and rejected by the body, unable to survive or achieve any useful function in a hostile and eventually lethal environment.

A great debate has arisen from the interesting evidence of the therapeutic potential of stem cells, and the ethical questions posed by obtaining the cells via human embryos (from the implantation of the blastocyst in the mucous membrane of the womb until the eighth week) or even foetuses (from the eighth week until birth). This has led to the governments of different countries seeking the guidance of scientists, bioethicists and judges to establish new rules to regulate the use of these cells, as wrongful trade could lead to criminal abortions in order to obtain them.

Although this is shaky ground, there is some agreement that the least problematic source of stem cells is the thousands of embryos that originate from assisted reproduction treatment which are kept frozen in liquid nitrogen.

Current legislation in some countries (Spain amongst them) only permits research on human embryos that are less than 14 days old, provided that they are not viable.

On the other hand, it is necessary to establish well-regulated guidelines on the maximum time during which the frozen embryo maintains its viability and potential intact, as the negative effects of prolonged freezing are already known. Frozen embryos (those obtained additionally during assisted reproduction) have existed in Spain for 15 years. In Great Britain it was ordered that embryos of a similar source, older than five years, should be destroyed, which provoked protests from the Catholic sectors. How long should they be kept frozen? What is the optimum freezing time? Why can we successfully freeze sperm and embryos and not ovules? Who is or who are the "owners" of these embryos? Should they be legally donated in order to be able to use them in scientific research?

It is evident that there are still numerous unknowns to clear up in this field and the suggestion that those committees instructed by various governments to study the multiple implications of this type of research ought to "prioritise research on stem cells of an animal origin", makes complete sense.

It is appropriate to recall here that a good number of discoveries made in the field of human fertility occurred as a consequence of research work on sheep, financed by the wool industry, especially in Australia.

There currently exists a "fashion" (as it is difficult to predict how long it will last) of freezing the blood from the removed umbilical cord of a newborn, in order to preserve the stem cells so that it may be used later in life by the same person, if required. Maintaining the blood at optimum freezing conditions comes at a high price. Here the same question arises regarding the time period of firm viability for the frozen cells, for if it is limited, as we currently think, then the blood will be of little use to its owner if they come to need it at the end of their life.

The procurement of foetal tissue, and the temptation of criminal abortions in order to obtain it, have diminished with the spread of the knowledge that what counts are the stem cells and that there exist other more convenient and less problematic sources.

At my request, Professor Karem Noris-Suárez has provided the following comments:

"The stem cells paradox doesn't end with deciding between embryonic or adult blood from the cryopreserved umbilical cord or stem cells from the bone marrow, autologous or donor. The great unknown is which is the true operating system. For scientific studies indicate that the function *in vivo* is that of regulating the immune system more than that of converting themselves into new functional cells . . . and to achieve this last one, support can only be achieved through the engineering of the tissues.

"The use of only stem cells does not bring great benefits if we think about them in isolation. The great goal for scientists at this time is to understand as a whole the environment that truly regulates those cells with their capacity for regeneration, and in parallel brings new cells that differ in their cellular functions under strict systems of control."

82nd Paradox
Birth control and family planning: Natural methods vs. Artificial contraceptive methods

By family planning I mean birth control via the employment of contraceptive methods designed to permit couples responsibly to decide the number of children they wish to have.

The natural method is based on symptoms suggestive of fertility in a woman: temperature and other minor symptoms (cervical mucus or the Billings method* published in 1970). When correctly practised it has a very high effectiveness, estimated by the World Health Organisation at around 98%.

The best-known method is the Ogino-Knaus method (simultaneously discovered by the Japanese doctor Kyusaku Ogino (1882–1975) and the Austrian doctor Hermann Knaus (1892–1970)), which is a natural method of birth control based on knowledge of a woman's fertile days. Specifying the day of ovulation (the basal temperature rises after ovulation due to progesterone which is secreted by the luteal body) and bearing in mind that the average life of an egg is only 24 hours and of sperm a little more than that, it is possible to calculate which days in the feminine ovulation cycle are fertile. By abstaining from sexual relations on the periovulatory days it is feasible to avoid pregnancy, without the help of artificial methods. Natural methods are the only ones accepted by the Catholic Church.

Other methods generatively denominated as "abortive" include any birth planning method, including the death of a recently formed embryo. They include, barrier methods (condom for men, diaphragm for women) and Karman's method (abortion during the first two weeks of amenorrhea via vacuum aspiration).

* So called in honour of its inventor the Catholic doctor Australian John Billings (1918–2007)

83rd Paradox
Theoretical medical training vs. Practical medical training

"Better a hands-on doctor than one well-read." (La Celestina)

In reality this has never really been a true paradox. From the beginning, at least since the second half of the Middle Ages, medicine and surgery, separated as different jobs, were based on a lengthy education at the side of a reputable teacher thus ensuring that after many years of day-to-day experience the trainee would develop practical skills in the role. In this detail our profession was no different to the other numerous jobs that emerged in medieval cities and which formed the trade unions or corporations ("guilds" in English) that are still maintained with their ancient traditions in London. In fact surgeons were originally part of the guild of barbers.

In that period the great difference between doctors and surgeons was based on the required theoretical training of doctors (very quickly picked up by the emerging universities), versus its almost total absence for the surgeon-barbers of the period.

I have always been struck by the excellent practical training of students of medicine during their formal university studies (in hospitals, external surgeries, dispensaries, clinics, rural medical centres, etc.), which I attribute to the powerful and logical medical tradition, in contrast with the absence of similar training in the real work of other liberal professions (law, engineering, etc.).

A careful balance between the solid theoretical and practical training of the doctor is a result of considerable age-old experience in medical studies beginning at Salerno Medical School, through to medical schools of note such as those of Paris and Montpellier in France, and St Thomas and St Bartholomew's in England,which even preceded the foundation of the two famous universities of Oxford and

Cambridge. Medical studies never forgot this hospital past and it is inconceivable that a medical student would not train at the bedside of a hospitalised patient, caring for them under the direct supervision of a qualified teacher. This same concept is applied to the study of nursing. It is concerning to observe repeated attempts to alter this balance, which has been proven over centuries, in favour of a more "chalk and blackboard" theoretical classroom-based training, which reduces costs but which can never replace practical teaching with a patient.

84th Paradox
Chemical control of the risk factors of myocardial infarction
and cerebrovascular accident vs. Treatment of already
established diseases

The statistics are convincing. Cardiovascular diseases (including cerebrovascular accidents or ictus) are the main cause of death in the United
States. It is estimated, at the time of writing, that there are 62 million
people (in a population of 280 million) with cardiovascular diseases and
50 million with hypertension. In the year 2000, 946,000 deaths, 39%
of all deaths, were due to this cause. There is an ever-present interest
in controlling this pre-dominant cause of morbidity and mortality.

Two professors of epidemiology at the University of London, Wald
and Law (Sir Nicholas Wald and Malcolm Law) recently published
the findings of research from a review of more than 750 clinical tests,
meta-analyses and cohort studies. The result is an innovative and ambitious preventative medicine concept that intends to prevent the group
of degenerative diseases most common in the mature adult and the
elderly, specifically myocardial ischemia and cerebrovascular accidents.

For those who complain, with some reason, of the lack of new
"medical miracles" in the last two decades, it will perhaps be a surprise
to read the editorial and three of the scientific works published in the
British Medical Journal (*BMJ*) on 28 June 2003, in which their authors
boldly claim that a preventative strategy for the aforementioned diseases constitutes, "a greater impact on the prevention of disease in the
Western world than any other known intervention". (Rodgers, 2003)

For his part Dr Richard Smith, the ex-editor of the *BMJ* (one of
the most reliable and reputable medical journals in the world) has
no hesitation in stating, "It's perhaps more than 50 years since we
published something as important as the cluster of papers from Nick

Wald, Malcolm Law, and others. They argue convincingly that a pill with six ingredients could prevent 80% of heart attacks (or other events caused by ischaemic heart disease) and strokes. Anybody with cardiovascular disease would take the pill, and so would everybody from 55 – without any investigation." (Smith, 2003)

As it concerns diseases that eventually kill or severely incapacitate half of the populations of developed countries, if the strategy proposed by the authors can be widely proven, we could in effect be in the presence of a new and promising "medical miracle".

If, as has happened in the past, the results do not fulfil the expectations of the aforementioned strategy, for example with hormonal replacement therapy in postmenopausal women, we will have further reason to suspect the statistical method employed.

The concept behind the proposed strategy is based on a rational and simple logic. If we know, as in effect we do, the principal risk factors of those two processes that affect the heart and the brain, and if we have pharmaceuticals that can control those factors and maintain them at normal levels, why not combine them in suitable doses (which are lower than those habitually prescribed), in order to prevent these diseases which are so widely spread amongst the over-55 generation.

This proposition, which in itself is simple, needed to be proven by a series of serious studies, such as those undertaken and now published by Professors Wald and Law who, given their experience and previous achievements, have a high degree of credibility in the scientific world.

The famous proposed "polypill" has six ingredients: a statin, three pharmaceuticals to lower blood pressure (a thiazide, a beta-blocker and an angiotensin-converting enzyme inhibitor, each one at half of the standard dose), folic acid and aspirin.

According to the authors, a third of people who take the polypill on a daily basis from the age of 55 will benefit from the treatment, gaining on average 11 years of life, supposedly free of heart attacks and strokes. The side effects are minor with symptoms presenting themselves in 8–15% of treated cases.

Can the critical factors upon which these diseases depend really be chemically regulated on a continual basis? Is this a new version of the "magic bullet" by Paul Ehrlich*?

The proposition is tempting and, according to the aforementioned scientific articles, economically viable, as the majority of the pill's ingredients' patents have expired. The ground is therefore fertile for a manufacturer of generic pharmaceutical products to produce the pill in great quantities and at a reasonable price.

Will these pharmaceuticals at the prescribed dosage maintain their therapeutic effect over years of continual administration?

Will there be no development of intolerance phenomena and side effects?

The alternative, which is to await the appearance of these diseases with their signs and symptoms and disagreeable and costly consequences, will cease to be an option as soon as the reliability of the strategy proposed by the British scientists is proven.

The magnitude and importance of the proposal means that I have no doubt that we will have more information in the short term and that the governments of sovereign nations and, undoubtedly, international health bodies will have to reach a decision about it, facilitating the distribution of the pill to populations older than 55 years old. For it is precisely this age group, let's say between 55 and 75 years old, that has a significant economic value to their nations, as when enjoying full health their work and experience are an important factor in the prosperity of a country.

* Paul Ehrlich (1854–1915), German doctor and scientist

As was to be expected, almost immediately comments rained down about the authors' claims in the aforementioned article (11 of them on 27/6/2003) via the "rapid response" system available on the *BMJ* website, the majority of which expressed serious doubts about the methodology employed. It is clear that the last word about this matter has not been had, and that many years will pass before we can objectively judge the validity and true significance of the proposed strategy. In the meantime, it is logical to suppose that it will cause serious controversy amongst those who favour and those who are riled by the said strategy.

On an anecdotal note, I cannot fail to recall the opinion of one of my dearest teachers at New York University about the end of life. When I went to visit the Venezuelan dermatologist Juan Larralde in hospital, where he was recuperating from a heart attack, I found him in very good spirits. Smiling, he told me the reason, "I already know which illness I'm going to die from, and it is the least bad of them all."

If its assumptions turn out to be valid, the foreseeable consequences of such a strategy could mean a greater average lifespan, and death in the elderly would mostly be caused by cancer and degenerative diseases of the central nervous system (for example, Parkinson's and Alzheimer's). Such a perspective is not very cheering given that in spite of the huge efforts undertaken we still do not have adequate answers to those problems.

85th Paradox
Hygieia vs. Asclepius

It is said, justifiably I believe, that there is nothing new under the sun, and the Ancient Greek myths of Hygieia and Asclepius and the "never-ending oscillation" between the different points of view in medicine that they represent is proof of this.

For followers of Hygieia, health is the natural order of things, the positive attribute of a wisely lived life. The main function of medicine is to discover and teach those natural rules that guarantee a healthy body and mind.

Followers of Asclepius (*Aesculapius* in Latin) believe that the essential role of medicine is to treat illness, that is to say to restore health by correcting any imperfection caused by accident of birth or acquired in life.

86th Paradox
Medical novels and medical suspense novels: Spread of information vs. Information distortion

Of the great medical novels, two have been awarded the Nobel Prize for Literature: Thomas Mann (1875–1955), German author of *The Magic Mountain*, was given this treasured recognition in 1929; and the American author of *Arrowsmith*, Sinclair Lewis (1885–1951), received the prize in 1930. Both novels are classics that reflect fundamental aspects of the relationship between medicine and society.

Another widely read work is the autobiography *The Story of San Michele* by the Swedish doctor Axel Munthe (1857–1949).

In more recent times, the Nobel Prize for Literature was awarded to José Saramago (1922–2010) for his classic novel *Blindness*, which alerted us to "the responsibility of having my eyesight when others have lost theirs" ... (Saramago, 2013: 238)

The veritable explosion in the new literary genre of medical suspense novels demonstrates the importance that contemporary society attaches to healthcare. The majority of these novels are written by practising doctors or by those who have at least practised medicine in the past. They describe in precise detail the doctor-patient relationship, the life of a doctor, their doubts and tribulations, diagnosis techniques and treatment of many illnesses, all of which contributes to the circulation of this type of information amongst the general public; information which in the not too distant past was rather mysterious and arcane.

The negative side of information being spread by these means is that the stories frequently involve doctors carrying out immoral or illegal acts, from which our profession, like any other, is not exempt although cases are undoubtedly in a scarce minority. However, such behaviour, even in fiction, can potentially establish a certain level of doubt about a doctor's conduct and motivations, which in the long term degrades and erodes a relationship that is based on credibility and trust.

I think that in general the balance is positive and the doctor is placed in the exalted position that they have always had in society, where their key role as a fundamental instrument of the preservation and restoration of the health of the ill human being is recognised; a situation to which we are all, without exception, exposed during our existential journey.

The most famous of all medical novelists is undoubtedly the Scottish author Sir Arthur Conan Doyle (1859–1930), creator of Sherlock Holmes – a character inspired by Dr Joseph Bell, his Professor at the University of Edinburgh Faculty of Medicine – and his faithful companion Dr Watson, whose adventures are described in 58 novels.

Contemporary medical novelists include the French author Jean Reverzy (1914–59), Americans Frank G. Slaughter (1908–2001), William Pomidor (1962–), Stephen Bergman (1944–), pen name Samuel Shem), Perri Klass (1958–), Robert Marion and the Egyptian Nawal El Saadawi (1931–).

As for medical suspense novels, this literary genre has recently flourished in the English-speaking world with its principal cultivators being medical-novelists like Robin Cook (1940–), Francis Roe (1932–) and Walt McConnell (1931–).

87th Paradox
Evidence-based medicine vs. Empiricism

Evidence-based medicine in founded on a practice that only accepts scientifically proven knowledge as the basis for clinical judgement, and rejects treatments that, even though they may be frequently applied, lack reasons to argue in their favour. Its growing influence is derived from the work of a group at the University of McMaster in Ontario, Canada, which was published in November 1992 in *The Journal of the American Medical Association (JAMA)*.

This approach is based on scientific medicine, which we understand to be medicine that is based on theoretical knowledge of man, his illnesses and the peculiarities of the healthy and ill organism; this focus of medicine dates back to Classical Greece. Evidence-based medicine is supported by randomised, double-blind clinical trials, designed to bring the objectivity that is absent from casuistic empirical observations.

Two decades ago the subject of evidence-based medicine, which has been defined as "the conscientious, explicit, and judicious use of current best evidence in making decisions about the care of individual patients" (Sackett, Rosenberg *et al*, 1996: 71–2), has become the subject of a heated debate on the opportunities it presents, its advantages and possible consequences.

By contrast, empiricism, as a philosophical theory, emphasises the role of experience, and yet the knowledge and the language in which it is expressed are interpretative, hence the emergence of a collective evaluation of the best validation mechanisms.

The correct instrument for the promotion and utilisation of evidence-based medicine is undoubtedly The Cochrane Collaboration. Initiated in 1993, this is a significant international cooperative endeavour,

215

independent and not-for-profit with 31,000 volunteers from more than 120 countries. It has created an independent network of health professionals, researchers and patients to respond to the challenge presented by the enormous quantity of research-generated evidence and its possible utility in health-related decisions. Its mission is to generate accessible systematic reviews, encouraging any decisions taken in the health sector to be based in proven evidence. The Cochrane Collaboration is named to honour Dr Archibald L. Cochrane (1909–88), the Scottish doctor who was a pioneer of this movement.

88th Paradox
Cancer treatment: Surgery vs. Radiotherapy vs. Chemotherapy

The cancer problem is much more complex than it was thought to be some years ago; however, after decades of public interest focused on the issue and multimillion-dollar investments, not only of economic resources but also of the most highly-qualified research human resources in that area, we can make a preliminary assessment of the current situation and what has been achieved.

Thousands of scientific evaluations of the main three methods of destroying cancerous cells, used in isolation or in different combinations, are published every year.

If we can make any prediction with a degree of certainty, it is that we will observe a dramatic increase in incidences of cancer in the next two decades as a direct consequence of the increase in the average age of the population.

On 25 February 2003 during the Wellcome Lecture at the Royal Society of Medicine in London, which is given in memory of Professor Robert H. S. Thompson, Dr Karol Sikora*, an authority on this material, made some interesting assertions and predictions. He claimed that the most promising progress would come from the rapidly growing knowledge of the molecular biology of cancer. With a better understanding of the clear objectives of new pharmaceuticals it would be possible to establish a specificity in treatment, which would no longer be empirical, general and relatively inefficient in its spanning of different kinds of cancer. This in turn would translate into greater selectivity, less toxicity and the possibility of more prolonged administration.

* Dr Karol Sikora, Professor of Cancer Medicine at Imperial College and Hammersmith Hospital in London

Minimal invasive surgery will reduce the necessity of organ resuscitation, thereby avoiding a compromise of the patient's survival.

Highly sophisticated computerised radiotherapy systems will permit precise radiation planning, limiting its action to the form and spread of the tumour.

It is likely that preventative cancer drugs to reduce the risks of genetic deterioration will be developed.

By monitoring genes in blood serum and finding fragments of deoxyribonucleic acid (DNA) with defined mutations, the development of a genetic "chip" that sends signals to the patient's personal computer and kickstarts an investigation to determine the type and location of the primary tumour in its most incipient phase, could be envisaged.

By the year 2020, chemotherapy will probably replace other treatments in the majority of cancers. Professor Sikora believes that cancer will come to be, as some tumours already are, a controllable chronic illness similar to diabetes and hypertension today. Patients will receive treatment in much more agreeable establishments, in attractive surroundings similar to hotels. Global franchises will emerge for this purpose, substituting for hospitals and using the Internet to pass on specific treatment plans and monitor their quality almost instantaneously.

89th Paradox
Family medicine vs. Community medicine

The name family medicine indicates an integral primary care system. In family medicine the doctor does not just see the patient for an initial consultation, but will also follow through any possible procedures by medical specialists, remaining responsible for their patient throughout.

It is the foundation of the National Health Service in Great Britain which has lent its efficient medical services to the entire population of the country since 1948, and which represents a real paradigm of medical attention in the whole world, as no distinction is made between patients of differing economic resources.

Community medicine derives from community, a concept defined by the German sociologist Ferdinand Tonnies (1855–1936) as "opposed to society, in order to describe a particular form of social grouping based on natural relationships (familial), which constitute an organic form of social existence. Communal living is based on customs, a language and common traditions and on blood relations, friendship and solidarity, and lies in very sentimental roots".

It's possible to also use the term in relation to human groups that live in similar economical conditions, for example, in humble areas, which are deprived of the minimum of basic services (drinking water and adequate sewage disposal).

In the second half of the twentieth century the phenomenon of "urbanisation" occurred, the irreversible displacement of the rural population to the major cities, in an often fruitless search for a minimum of services, education, medical care and paid work. In Venezuela, the rate of urbanisation supersedes 90%. A large part of the population live on the periphery of big cities in precarious conditions, living in shanty towns (or shacks, huts, and *favelas*) which are unsafe and lacking in minimum hygiene conditions (i.e. lacking basic services like drinking water and sewage disposal). It is precisely in these places that a large part of the social unrest that seriously threatens the political stability of entire nations incubates, and which, with the different types of difficulties that it brings, tests the democratic governmental system.

In Caracas these communities are very obvious and visible as they are located in the hills that surround the stretch of valley where the centre of the city is located. Schemes designed to bring adequate medical assistance to these humble communities have not been particularly effective, which has recently led to a new social and political programme in Venezuela called *Barrio Adentro*. This scheme employs thousands of Cuban doctors who are contractually obliged to live in said areas, supposedly adopting the role of "family doctors". The effectiveness of this project is yet to be proven; however, there already exists a strong opposition to it, in particular from the medical profession, suspicious that the "importation" of these doctors has a strong political undertone whereby the Cuban physicians play an important role of political indoctrination of the more needy and humble population to whom they are supposed to provide decent medical care.

90th Paradox
Human medicine vs. Technical medicine

The problem of the dehumanisation of medicine in post-industrial society is universal. It is clearly linked to the great technological advances achieved in the twentieth century, which have tempted those who have mastered certain techniques to depend on them to an extreme, and at times exclusive, extent. This has led to the shunting to one side of what we have been taught ad nauseam since Hippocrates at the dawn of scientific medicine, and those other perspectives aforementioned in various other paradoxes in this book.

As the surgeon Atul Gawande* appreciates: "The core predicament of medicine – the thing that makes being a patient so wrenching, being a doctor so difficult, and being a part of society that pays the bills they run up so vexing – is uncertainty. With all that we know nowadays about people and diseases and how to diagnose and treat them, it can be hard to see this, hard to grasp how deeply uncertainty runs. As a doctor, you come to find, however, that the struggle in caring for people is more often with what you do not know than what you do. Medicine's ground state is uncertainty. And wisdom – for both the patients and doctors – is defined by how one copes with it." (Gawande, 2002: 229)

By accepting this view, it becomes quite clear that the human part of medical practice dominates the technical part.

---

* Atul Gawande (1965–), American surgeon, journalist and writer

91st Paradox
The patient's decision vs. The treating doctor's decision

In *Complications: A Surgeon's Notes on an Imperfect Science*, the American surgeon Atul Gawande (previously mentioned in Paradox 90) discusses the recent radical change in his country in the level of information provided to patients by their treating doctors. This is especially the case in establishing who bears the responsibility for taking decisions about which treatment to follow, particularly when it comes to surgical interventions.

He says that barely two decades ago, doctors made the decisions and patients obediently followed their prescribed treatment. Occasionally, if they had serious doubts, they would get a second opinion, that is to say, "the result of the patient's consultation of a second doctor with the object of confirming the diagnosis or prognosis of the first. To obtain it, the patient usually seeks the results of analyses and tests carried out by the first doctor and it is often this that raises the doctor's suspicion, unfounded if their activity was correct, given that the patient is only trying to be more certain. For this reason the request for the clinical history must be carried out with the greatest tact and courtesy on the part of the patient, and the doctor that receives the request for a second opinion must abstain from criticising their colleague although their technical opinion may differ." Gawande refers us to the fact that until a few years ago, "Doctors did not consult patients about their desires and priorities, and routinely withheld information – sometimes crucial information – such as what drugs they were on, what treatments they were being given, and what their diagnosis was. Patients were even forbidden to look at their own medical records: it wasn't their property, doctors said. They were regarded as children: too fragile and simple-minded to handle the truth, let alone make decisions. And they suffered for it. People were put on machines, given drugs, and subjected to operations they would not have chosen. And they missed out on treatments that they might have preferred." (Gawande, 2002: 210)

Suddenly everything changed. Part of the reason for this substantial turnabout was the appearance of the book *The Silent World of the Doctor and Patient* by University of Yale doctor, Jay Katz (1922–2008), a devastating criticism of the doctor/patient decision making process which undoubtedly had a great influence on the change that occurred.

Perhaps the pendulum has moved excessively in the opposite direction, as currently the predominant custom in the United States is to unload the entire wealth of information and statistics on to the patient and their family, without committing to one direction or another, leaving the patient to make the decision on their own.

On reading this paradox my son, Francisco A. Kerdel (who is a doctor) commented, justifiably I believe: "Nor can we wash our hands like Pontius Pilate and leave the patient to make the decision on their own." Understanding the patient permits the doctor to win his or her confidence and ensure that the doctor's advice is followed.

92nd Paradox
Allopathic medicine vs. Homeopathic medicine

Allopathy (from the Greek *állos* meaning different and *páthos* meaning suffering) was the term coined by the German doctor Samuel Hahnemann (1755–1843) to describe the focus of orthodox medicine, which prescribes medication to suppress symptoms of an illness utilising the principle of opposites (for example analgesics for pain, purgatives for constipation), in contrast to the system he invented called homeopathy, which favours rather than antagonises the body's reactions to the illness process.

Since the introduction of homeopathy in the nineteenth century, the medical orthodox has considered it a form of alternative medicine, "which seeks to cure like with like; instead of attacking the cause of the illness through an antagonist product, very small doses of products that provoke the same symptoms of the illness that you wish to treat should be prescribed. According to homeopathic theory, the organism will react against these micro doses, repelling the illness and reaching a cure on its own. Its efficacy has been proven in numerous cases, veterinary homeopathy also exists and is effective. However, its mechanism of action is unknown and there are many opportunists who practise it without having studied in depth the little of what is understood about it." (Universidad de Navarra, 2000)

93rd Paradox
Medical novels vs. Medical autobiographies

It is important to distinguish between novels with medical subject matter, whose principal characters are generally doctors (and are sometimes written by doctors), and autobiographical works, whose authors are doctors. In the first case it's a matter of fiction, in the second real memories.

These days, even authors with no medical background can write a medical novel or a novel with medical characters. These authors, whose profession by its very nature creates the expectation of a certain artistic licence in fiction, spend months, even years, researching in order to accurately position the action in the environment that they describe, ensuring that, in particular, the dialogue in anything related to medicine is as close to reality as possible.

The result of the contemporary novelist's self-imposed "responsibility" to research areas of specialised knowledge is that the reader takes the novels very seriously, assuming in good faith that what appears printed in black and white is what happens in reality, or at least in reality as interpreted by the author of the book they are reading (or hear on the radio or see on television). It is undoubtedly a very important element in informing the general public of what medicine is and what doctors in today's society represent.

Medical novels are also a valuable source of information and inspiration for young secondary students aspiring to study medicine, or those people seriously contemplating medical studies. These people understandably wish to familiarise themselves with the type of life offered to them by a profession that involves out of the ordinary obligations and which demands a level of dedication, sacrifice even, which is uncommon in other areas.

Reading this type of fiction at a crucial time in our lives, when we are still young and permeable to that type of influence, can determine whether medicine is the profession to which we wish to dedicate the rest of our lives.

I recall reading of the influence that the book *Microbe Hunters* by Paul de Kruif* had for many years on people aspiring to study medicine. I cannot help but remember nostalgically the first time I read the book, published in 1926, which describes the great achievements of those responsible for the discovery of the causative agents of infectious and contagious diseases, of the vectors of some of those endemics, and some of their treatments. The book has chapters dedicated to Antonie van Leeuwenhoek (1632–1723), the first "microbe hunter"; Lazzaro Spallanzani (1729–99); Louis Pasteur (1822–95); Robert Koch (1843–1910); Émile Roux (1853–1933); Emil von Behring (1854–1917); Ilya Metchnikoff (1845–1916); Theobald Smith (1859–1934); Sir David Bruce (1855–1931); Sir Ronald Ross (1857–1932); Giovanni Battista Grassi (1954–25); Walter Reed (1851–1902); and Paul Ehrlich (1854–1915). My teacher Dr Humberto García Arocha gave it to me as a prize for biology when I was studying the fourth year of my high school diploma at the Liceo Andrés Bello in Caracas; it undoubtedly contributed to my decision to pursue a career in medicine.

In his simple style, Kruif recounts the veritable epic of the "microbe hunters" who, with the exception of the first two, achieved the incredible feat of establishing the aetiology of microbial and parasitic illnesses in the second half of the nineteenth century; they were precursory and indispensable discoveries to the therapeutic progress that would occur just a century later.

* Paul de Kruif (1890–1971), American bacteriologist and pathologist

94th Paradox
Fighting death vs. Assisting death

One of the greatest challenges faced by medicine across the most dissimilar of cultures and civilisations is deciding when to cease the fight for the patient's life and resign ourselves to accept death as the final destination of this transitory and fragile phenomenon called life.

We are already aware of the way in which the position of the contemporary doctor in relation to the definition of death has changed from the age-old view of death as the cessation of heartbeat and respiratory movement (as their functions can be artificially maintained), to brain death, or neocortical death, and the difficulties of establishing it.

A death diagnosis is defined as "the irreversible cessation of bodily functions as a whole, assessed by the symptoms that produce the cessation of functions. Given that the symptoms take time to exhibit, they cannot be identified with mathematical accuracy, and there will be a few minutes in which resuscitation techniques may be tried in the notion that even though a cardiac arrest has occurred, the body may not yet have reached an irreversible situation." (Universidad de Navarra, 2000)

If used irrationally, current technological developments can lead to therapeutic over-zealousness, using "therapies that cannot cure the patient, but simply prolong their life in painful conditions". (Clínica Universidad de Navarra, 2015) This final stage of life can lead to a do-not-resuscitate order, "which appears in the patient's clinical history so that in the case of cardiac arrest neither the nursing team nor the emergency doctor try revival manoeuvres and instead let the patient die. It is employed in cases where it is positively known that said manoeuvres would constitute therapeutic obstinacy or would be futile." (Universidad de Navarra, 2000)

But the problem does not just lie in these sometimes justified, sometimes desperate attempts to resuscitate a patient, but rather in today's prevailing, perhaps subconscious, irrational resistance to accepting death as a final and definitive biological fact, a law to which we are all subject, without exception, all living organisms, from single cells to man in his immense structural and functional complexity.

This leads to our unjustified feeling that natural death is a failure, or at least a fault, of medicine. This is completely absurd as nobody is more familiar than medical staff with the transition from life to death and its irreversibility; a thought that we push to one side, on an individual and personal level, throughout our lives.

This situation undoubtedly derives from the fact that many diseases end in death (all too frequently premature death, if we take into account current life expectancy), and that death in some cases can be attributed to medical malpractice, including surgical errors and complications, or in other words, from the intervention of a doctor or doctors.

The practice of gerontology must be hard, having to continually contend with the gradual deterioration of the body until death is inevitably reached.

Every doctor, according to his or her age, speciality and experience, will have faced this painful and complex situation, and will have formed an opinion about it. For this reason it is appropriate to include here extracts from the memoirs and essays of colleagues about those feelings awakened by their experiences with death:

Pedro Lain Entralgo:
Is death medicine's horizon? The doctor tries to avoid it, but as soon as an illness escalates and they are faced with the imminent possibility of death, when they see that they are powerless to stop the progressive extinction of life, when they have been frequently exposed to the risk

and imminence of death, they understand that the death of a patient is medicine's unavoidable horizon. Today more than ever, it is necessary to teach doctors what death is; human death needs to be understood. In this respect we have to distinguish between the fact, the act and the event of death. The fact: what really happens in the human body during its passing. The act: what the dying person does when they feel and think that they will inevitably die soon. The event: what happens socially as a consequence of the death of a person. All of this matters to the doctor, and very little about it is said to him.

Fernando Serpa Flores:
Those long years of sustained effort concluded, the intern . . . with long wakeful nights facing death, who cynically brandishes her scythe before our eyes, as if wanting to tell us that we wasted our time studying how to fight her, for she, at the end of the day, would always win.

Only after years of contemplating suffering do we reach an understanding that this respectable enemy is loyal and wise. It is difficult to achieve, but imperceptibly, like one who enjoys making their lover suffer, we gradually come to understand her hidden charms. My first friendly encounter with death occurred in the least expected place, and the first time that I called to her in peace, recognising that perhaps due to my inexperience and carried by the vanity of my arrogance, I had not had the opportunity to appreciate her qualities. In a *hospital of the fallen*, in a leper's hospital, sharing the pain of our mutilated and blind brothers, I raised a silent prayer to death asking for her pardon for my incomprehension of her . . .

*   *   *

Accepting with good grace what death means is impossible for the great majority of human beings, indeed past and present religions are founded on the great mystery that it represents.

But, there is a great distance between understanding and accepting death and actively contributing to her acceleration, as attempted by euthanasia or "assisted suicide".

One has to make a distinction here with "suicide assistance". Suicide assistance is defined as "a medical contribution to the suicide of a patient, generally providing medicine in the sufficient dosage to provoke a painless death. It is different from euthanasia in that the doctor does not personally administer said means. Paradoxically, its practice does not bring about the suicide of the patient in the majority of cases, but instead brings the tranquillity of knowing that if their illness worsens they will have the means at hand. A request for assisted suicide on the part of the patient usually reveals suffering that has been inadequately treated. Doctors are often scared (unjustifiably so) to prescribe morphine; skimping on it is a very common error, which only causes unhelpful suffering."

On the other hand, we understand helping people to die as "the doctor's care in the last moments of a patient's life. Including the palliative care necessary for their physical relief (pain, discomfort) and the support and moral comfort required (company, calming worries, religious assistance)."

In relation to this final role of the doctor, when consolation and moral support for the patient and their closest relatives is required, it is necessary to coordinate what happens with the family, any religious representatives (if the patient is a believer) and even organisations established for this purpose, (such as "The Natural Death Movement" in Great Britain), which creates a parallel between the birth and the death of a person, supporting the idea that the patient prefers to die in their own home accompanied by their family and close friends, than in the cold dehumanised, anonymous environment of a big hospital. There is even the suggestion of a new role, a specialist in calming the anxiety brought on by the proximity of death, the equivalent of what a midwife represents at a birth. It is a nascent idea that may develop and end up playing an important social function. On the www.globalideasbank.org website there is an interesting disquisition about "brave and conscious deaths" of exceptional historical characters, with details on the last moments of men and women whose examples are a model for the rest of the human race.

95th Paradox
Managed health care systems vs. Fees for services rendered

The traditional payment system for doctors is fees for services rendered.

According to the *Diccionario Espasa de Medicina*, fees are "money received by the doctor or any liberal professional in general for the practice of their profession. The word fees refers to the fact that more than pay, said money is a reward for the honour that their careful dedication to others deserves: medical attention and money are disproportionate, money is inadequate to measure the value of medical attention".

In this sense medicine is radically divorced from the other liberal professions (law, engineering, architecture, etc.), as their fees are not based on the patient's economic prowess or an estimate of the economic value of the service rendered, but instead on the complexity or difficulty of the service provided. These days more than ever, the majority of medical cases are regulated by indexes or rates of precisely fixed remunerations for each medical or surgical procedure, and are established by non-medical third parties – generally insurance companies.

Health maintenance organisations, commonly called HMOs, have their roots in non-profit organisations, such as Kaiser Permanente, which from the 1930s was one of the first institutions to offer pre-paid medical services. The conceptual, philosophical basis of the system is the theory that it is more economical to pay for medical service continuously, where the physician has a material interest in maintaining the good health of their client, and where if the client becomes ill the costs of treating their poor health will already be included in the premium that they pay on a regular basis. Therefore no additional costs are involved and the institution has a real financial interest in looking out for the good health of their members. The central idea of paying a regular moderate sum to ensure that you remain healthy and with no incurring of additional costs when you become unwell is clearly attractive to the general public. Moreover, two activities that were previously divorced – medical insurance and medical attention – are combined in the same institution, which in theory makes them more effective.

As you can imagine, things are not as simple as they first appear. In practice HMOs have become distorted to the extent that they have become the powerful profit-making institutions that are progressively taking over medical care in many countries.

This distortion happened in stages. When in the '70s, the costs related to medical care in the United States grew much more quickly than the rest of the economy, it was thought that the fee system for services rendered was one of the causes, as doctors had no incentive to try to control costs. In order to reduce these costs, in 1973 Richard Nixon's administration put forward to Congress the Health Maintenance Organization Act, which created the term HMO. This required businesses with more than 25 employees to offer HMO cover to their employees, if they already offered them standard insurance. The law awarded federal funds to assist the start up of HMOs during the development period. The term HMO was coined by Dr Paul Ellwood (1926–), health consultant to Nixon, in order to describe the combination of insurance and medical care in the same organisation.

In 1974, American Congress approved the Employee Retirement Income Security Act (or ERISA) in order to protect HMOs from the majority of malpractice claims.

By the end of the 1970s HMOs were a much reduced part of the American health care system, enrolling just 5% of the population. That participation grew 400% in a decade, from 9 million in 1980 to 36 million in 1990. In 1987, 27% of employees were incorporated in an HMO, and by 1996 the figure had increased to 74%.

The majority of Americans are enrolled in profit-making HMOs, like Aetna or Cigna. These organisations represent 75% of HMO plans (an increase from the 18% that they represented in 1981).

The capitalisation of HMO businesses, into publically registered companies of this type whose shares are traded on the stock exchange, grew from 3.3 billion dollars in 1987 to 38.9 billion by the end of 1997.

According to the WHO, the health expenditure per capita in the United States was USD 8,608 in 2011, and this cost as a percentage of GDP grew to 17.9%.

96th Paradox
Medical ethos vs. General cultural ethos*

The favoured hypothesis suggested throughout this book is that medical studies and later medical practice itself, for good or bad, firmly influence a doctor's way of being, behaving and understanding life. We can therefore justify our attempts in this work to view the literary and scientific production of the doctor as the establishment of a common denominator, which is influenced to a certain extent by the medical "ethos" that marks out the initiated of this profession. For this reason I have attempted to isolate, identify and distinguish the creativity of the doctor as a singular product that is worthy of being studied separately and judged by its own merits. Perhaps it would be a little radical to claim that those who have only vaguely been involved in medicine for a short time have "infected" or "contaminated" (according to the viewpoint with which they are observed) such a peculiar "ethos", but it is undoubtedly a factor that we cannot easily put to one side.

If we can conceive of an "ethos" that is particular to every segment of culture, then medicine is undoubtedly it.

The medical history scholar easily establishes the existence of individuals who were not doctors but who had a great curiosity in the human body, as well as medicine, for example Leonardo da Vinci (1452–1519) who possibly mastered human anatomy better than the medical graduates of his era. Therefore this medical ethos is most certainly shared by intellectuals who are deeply interested in the serious study of the human body and the illnesses that affect it, and this establishes

* Ethos is a Greek word meaning "character" used to describe the beliefs and ideals that characterise a community, nation or ideology.

a certain methodology, which is then reflected in any type of creative work by the doctor, particularly literary work. This is a debatable but possible, even probable, proposition.

97th Paradox
Famous doctors as doctors vs. Famous doctors in other disciplines

The history of the cultural universe permits us to identify great men (and women) whose creativity and genius was developed in the terrain of the medical profession chosen by them. Such is the case with Hippocrates, Galen, Avicenna, Averroes, Maimonides, Vesalius, Harvey, etc.

However, there exists a large number of doctors who having excelled in areas outside of medicine are not identified as doctors by posterity. Their creativity, behaviour, actions and achievements perhaps cause it to be forgotten that medical training contributed, at least partially, to the original contributions that have given form and content to our culture.

Included in this group of famous doctors in other disciplines are: St Luke the Apostle (first century, religion), Nicolaus Copernicus (1473–1543, astronomy), John Locke (1632–1704, philosophy), Carl Linnaeus (1707–78, botany), Jean Paul Marat (1743–93, politics), Cesare Lombroso (1835–1909, criminology) and Henry Dunant (1828–1910, philanthropy).

98th Paradox
Human surgery vs. Robotic surgery

The impressive growth of the power of computing, measured by Moore's Law* establishes that computer chips are developing at an exponential rate. In fact, these improvements multiply and double in efficiency every two years, meaning that in the last forty years microprocessors have become millions of times more effective, which has numerous important implications for the health sector.

The three most exceptional advances permitted by this growth are: remote control surgery, keyhole surgery and robotic surgery.

Robotic surgery has become firmly established in the last few years, and its noted advantages include its precision, reduced incisions, fewer haemorrhages, less pain and shorter recuperation time.

Here we are limited to speculating on what may occur in the future, using Jaron Lanier's† vision in his now famous book *Who Owns the Future?*:

"Nanorobots, holographic radiation, or just plain old robots using endoscopes might someday perform heart surgery. These gadgets would perform the economic role that mp3 players and smartphones took on in music delivery. Whatever the details, surgery would then be reconceived as an information service. The role of human surgeons in that case is not predetermined, however. They will remain *essential*, for the technology will rely on data that has to come from people . . ." (Lanier, 2013: 7)

---

* Moore's Law established by Gordon E. Moore (1929–), says that according to the history of computing hardware, the number of transistors in integrated circuits doubles approximately every two years.
† Jaron Lanier (1960–)American writer, computer scientist and classical music composer

99th Paradox

The challenge of primary health care:

Traditional clinics vs. Cuban programme *Barrio Adentro*

By primary health care we mean "non-specialised medical attention which constitutes the first rung of attention for the patient in State health care systems". (*Diccionario España Medicina*)

In 2003 the Venezuelan government chose to create a dual system of primary health care, giving strong economic support to a new programme devised and planned in Cuba with the mission name *Barrio Adentro*, whilst maintaining existing clinics in a marginal way.

The Cuban communist revolutionary ideologists did not forget their objectives when they focused on the medical care sector, for apart from the evident importance of the links generated by the first contact between the doctor and the patient, it is generally accepted that around 80% of the illnesses discussed in a primary medical consultation are cured without medical intervention. This means guaranteed therapeutic success on entry, for no matter what medicine is prescribed the symptoms will disappear on their own in a few days, and the patient will always attribute their recovery to that prescription and the physician's professional expertise.

Possibly on the basis of this, the Cubans organised a large-scale fast track system of clearly incomplete medical training, and perhaps when they realised that they did not have the domestic market for the quantity of doctors that they had trained they resolved to export them, taking great care that it would seem like a gesture of international altruism, when in reality they had turned that supposed cooperation into human trade thereby permitting the island's government to balance their budget. There are numerous reports on this, but as an example let's take a newspaper piece from 5 February 2014, which describes the case of a Cuban doctor who joined the Brazilian *Más Médicos* programme launched by the Brazilian government in 2013 (similar to *Barrio Adentro*, but which sends Cuban doctors to remote rural areas in Brazil). This doctor declared that he received only US$400 per month, despite the agreement between Brazil and Cuba which established a monthly salary of US $4,166.

Undoubtedly the Cuban regime is making a lucrative business out of this mass exportation of doctors and it will have been an important motivation for the establishment of *Barrio Adentro* as the sending of Cuban doctors to Venezuela is largely offset by the daily delivery of one hundred thousand barrels of Venezuelan oil to Cuba.

According to *Wikipedia*, the *Barrio Adentro* mission is "a social programme, with the help of the Cuban government, characterised by the use of Cuban and Venezuelan doctors to offer health services to the Venezuelan population in the poor zones of the country (called barrios), in small clinics built and equipped with medical supplies in inaccessible areas which are far from hospitals." (12 June 2015)

A short time ago I read the book *Revolutionary Doctors* by the American author Steve Brouwer; a veritable apology for the Cuban medical training and care system, and absent of any negative criticism of a programme of which the validity, usefulness and stability are yet to be proven.

One has to take into account the current neglect of units and desertion by numerous Cuban doctors when considering the initial enthusiasm for the programme.

100th Paradox
Traditional doctors vs. Primary community physicians

As already mentioned in Paradox 24, educational innovations are highly risky as it takes years for their results to be realistically, definitively and convincingly established. If the results are negative, they have the potential to irreversibly affect many people, sometimes a whole generation, before the necessary corrections can be introduced.

Therefore, amongst other multiple and well-founded reasons, the Venezuelan government's initiative of introducing a parallel system of medical education, which is based on the simplified Cuban system, and attempting to equate it to the traditional system of medical education is undoubtedly an improvisation. Moreover, its consequences have the potential to create confusion and serious faults in the health system of the country, the likes of which are already being observed.

There is a long tradition of medical studies in Venezuela, initiated some 250 years ago during the colonial period, specifically 1763, when the Majorcan doctor Lorenzo Campins y Ballester (1726–85) obtained the necessary permission from the King of Spain to begin medical studies at what was then the Real y Pontificia Universidad de Caracas (founded in 1721 and currently the Universidad Central de Venezuela). Medicine has been taught in its classrooms, libraries, laboratories and affiliated hospitals since then, with the periodic incorporation of new knowledge and techniques to its teaching systems, such as the contributions of José María Vargas (1786–1854) at the beginning of the Republican era. After graduating in medicine in Caracas, José María Vargas studied for a postgraduate degree in medicine (ophthalmology, anatomy, pathology) and other subjects like mineralogy, botany and chemistry at the famous University of Edinburgh. On his return to Caracas in 1825 he was named Professor of Anatomy, and in 1827, Dean of the Universidad Central de Venezuela, the first doctor to achieve this elevated academic position, from where he was able to introduce many changes to modernise those institutions. In 1835 he became the first civilian president of the nascent republic, albeit for a short time only.

The example set by Vargas of travelling abroad to perfect the knowledge acquired in Venezuela and then returning to the country to apply it, has been followed since then to the present day by successive generations of doctors, first to Europe, mainly Paris, and then from the Second World War onwards, to the United States. This has allowed Venezuelan doctors to maintain a very high and up-to-date scientific level, updated by the contributions of each new generation of doctors.

Any assessments already made of Primary Community Physicians indicate that they leave much to be desired. It is quite clear why this short, improvised and deficient academic training by teachers with little experience – and therefore as improvised as their own training – produces such a different result.

"The Cuban trading company 'Comercializadora de Servicios Médicos Cubanos' is the intermediary company that sends off doctors, and is paid cash on delivery at one thousand dollars for each professional transferred, of which the doctor only receives 400 . . . The Cuban writer Carlos Montaner referred to Cuban doctors as "modern slaves": "They are the preferred slaves of the Comandante: he hires them, he sells them, he lends them out, he exchanges them for oil, he uses them as an excuse to justify his dictatorship."

If the problem really is that the number of health professionals needs to increase, then there are other better-tested solutions, such as "Medicaid" in the United States, which carries out some medical procedures, but always under the watchful eye and control of a qualified doctor.

EPILOGUE

Let me conclude by expressing once more the happiness, fulfilment and fortune I feel in having chosen medicine as my profession, and in having consistently and enthusiastically dedicated myself to this science and ancient and noble art. Many people in my family have chosen medicine as a profession: my maternal grandfather, two maternal uncles, my eldest son, my grandson, my brother, two brothers-in-law, a nephew, two first cousins (one paternal, one maternal), and one of their children. Five generations of doctors could be called "a medical dynasty" (which was not uncommon in the old countries of Europe: Jean Civatte, a professor of dermatology in Paris, for example, is the ninth generation of doctors in his family). If nepotism or influence-peddling in this respect is a concern, I recall a report on medical education commissioned by British parliament, which found that no opportunism had been found in the admission of the children of doctors into British schools of medicine. In reference to this finding, an MP (who was not a doctor) pointed out that even if it were the case, they would not perceive it to be a negative factor, as the children of doctors would be likely to have a more realistic idea of what medicine actually involves; something that is in fact equally removed from its two opposing visions, that of a preaching (quasi religious) view in the one extreme and a lucrative business in the other.

And, if as well as enjoying your job, you are convinced, as I always have been, that your work is helping to improve the quality of life of your patients, and that you can also spread your knowledge and experience to your fellow man through teaching and publishing, helping them to rid themselves of illness, prevent illness from occurring, and thereby enjoy better health, frankly I cannot think of anything that can successfully compete with this; choosing what we want to do and fulfilling this choice with a role of undoubted utility and benefit, in the thorough fulfilment of the journey that destiny has assigned to us.

QUO VADIS MEDICINE?

The study of the dilemmas, contradictions and paradoxes of current medicine necessarily leads us to attempt a diagnosis of its present situation and consider the possible corrections of the direction medicine is taking as a liberal profession in a short-term foreseeable future. Attempting a diagnosis of medicine's direction in the medium and long term is a futile intellectual exercise as it is practically impossible to achieve this with any degree of credibility, given the magnitude and significance of the changes to be expected.

Medicine currently relies on support from external sources, not only from the foundation science and technology sectors, but also an imposed administrative sector, which doctors continue to ignore as outside their professional practice. As long as this situation endures, where medicine remains completely dependent on external talent and creativity (something which is greater at times than others), the sense of frustration and uncertainty about the future of our profession will persist to a certain degree. Moreover, politicians (the most disgraced class of our era) have no hesitation in making demagogic and populist promises in this sector, thinking up ill-conceived programmes that are impossible to adequately carry out. Understanding very well the importance attributed to health by the electorate, they are only concerned in obtaining the majority vote in the next elections.

This affects the credibility of medicine and doctors, for in this irresponsible and messy confusion, establishing who is to blame is very difficult and politicians always manage to find a scapegoat for any failures. The public is therefore unable to discern whether the original unrealistic objective has been fulfilled.

This will most certainly be the final destination of the Chavez administration's *Barrio Adentro* programme, with its so-called doctors imported from Cuba who bring the practice of medicine to the most impoverished neighbourhoods in the hills surrounding Caracas and other cities in the country. In addition to their services as doctors, they also provide "Cubanised" Marxist indoctrination, the kind that follows the Fidel model (an idiosyncratic tropical Caribbean hybrid). In the end, the programme will be remembered as the government looking after that sector of society's medical needs, although they will resent being treated by foreign doctors of doubtful scientific training, who are more interested in political preaching than in their bodily or emotional well-being.

At the end of the day, it is men and women outside of the profession itself who are deciding the future of medicine, its objectives, difficulties, and traditions, indeed its very essence. Can we trust this and think for one moment that they will adopt those ideas and principles that have shaped medicine since the time of Hippocrates? Let us admit from the start that this is rather improbable and that doctors are understandably untrusting and cautious of accepting the supposedly curative prescriptions for the health system's complex problems, which are cooked up behind our backs, as a miracle cure.

Consequently, it is desirable that doctors should specialise in the basic areas of science, especially biology, genetics, immunology, biostatistics and pharmacology, where the most relevant and productive niches of research in the immediate future are to be found. This is equally the case in hybrid disciplines like bioengineering, hospital administration, etc., which should be incorporated without doubt or delay into well-structured departments in faculties of medicine. This way, at least some of the creativity, innovations and discoveries in these areas will come from the heart of where the knowledge is taught to those who aspire to be doctors. Even if most of this knowledge has other sources of origin, if its comprehension, adaption and utilisation occur in an intelligent, reasonable and clear way, a suitable voice for the new tonalities and rhythms of the research effort will be found at the heart of the medical teaching body.

On the other hand, given the maturity of the gigantic and multifaceted health industry – which has been built rather hastily and with little previous experience – both the medical profession and faculties of medicine need to dedicate time and effort to achieving a better understanding of the profession's "market" relations and to influencing directly new corporate schemes that offer greater and better participation to doctors, as the key players in the whole care process.

Both of these aspects are truly critical to the medical profession, as much for its growing future and development (scientific research), as its intricate economic relationship with the society that it serves. But it will only be possible to maintain medicine's pre-eminence if it employs the most gifted, suitably trained and informed staff, who are alert and adaptable to the changes that continually present themselves in an ever-increasing dynamic.

All of this represents a great challenge for schools of medicine, and demonstrates the incapacity of the medical profession to take on the new fields provided by the current evolution of human ingenuity, which is certain to grow exponentially in the future. This incapacity needs to change in order for medical knowledge to be generated and put it into practice. "*Laissez faire, laissez passer*", is a recipe for certain continual downturn, attrition and the future extinction of medicine, at least medicine as we know it, as a discipline that has developed successfully through history over the last two and a half uninterrupted millennia.

Attempting to understand these changes and prepare the necessary human resources within medicine's own structures to play an active role in the driving of these changes seems to be the most pertinent strategy in a moment of great worldwide turbulence, during which new systems of collective administration within health services are tested.

But before touching upon the issue of the incorporation of new disciplines – including the creation of hybrid disciplines within schools of medicine – we must turn our attention, albeit very briefly, to the importance of attracting to medical studies the most brilliant students with the most promising future in present and future generations. We must focus an intelligent effort on relaying to our colleges and high schools a very clear, optimistic, even enthusiastic, message about the opportunities and challenges of medicine in the future. Until recent years, the medical profession did not have any problems in this respect; indeed it was the preferred profession of secondary school students in every new generation of young people, and the medical school selection process guaranteed the recruitment of the most brilliant and promising students. Recent studies, from different sources and different countries, appear to indicate that the pendulum has started to move in the opposite direction. The young appear to have other professional careers in their sights, whether due to intellectual or physical laziness (long, costly and demanding studies and professional practice) or whether they perceive the problems currently facing medicine in crisis. Making them see with complete objectivity the opportunities and challenges of medicine in the future is the best strategy to follow, provided that the message is spread by leaders who are enlightened, motivated, enthusiastic, convincing, and above all brilliant. This is a collective task for the great schools of medicine. Given the advance of globalisation, we must recruit convincing and persuasive leaders, intellectual seducers if you like, from the international arena to pass on this universal message.

248

There must be must a well-considered plan of action and progressive implementation in order for new seats, departments and divisions in hybrid disciplines to be created, which will establish bridges and interrelations with other areas of knowledge whose development it is presumed will directly affect future medical practice.

If we start from the premise that the most gifted young people, men and women, are simultaneously the most ambitious from an intellectual point of view, we immediately understand that it is undoubtedly the great question marks and unresolved debates, challenges if you will, that most captivate and attract those restless minds of great potential who are seeking an appropriate path. It is not, therefore, the magnitude and complexity of the problem that discourages these young people from choosing medicine as the centre of their intellectual activity, but instead the lack of a clear and decisive message from our current natural leaders, who are rather perplexed and indecisive about which road to take.

The antiquity and importance of medical tradition, a vital characteristic for our profession, makes it an almost impossible obstacle to overcome for those forces attempting to convert medical practice into a mere exercise of sophisticated technology. This separates the interests of the generation that provided the knowledge to inspire said technology, from the inventiveness of the same and from its administration in the society that it serves. Doctors have long been the main characters in the health sector drama, and sharing that status takes time to accept. In view of the growth and complexity of health sciences, within which medicine is just one more actor, it is advisable from every point of view to try to understand what happens in medicine's neighbour disciplines, which nourish the knowledge and technologies that until now were considered our undisputed territory, well-demarcated by tradition. Hence the resentment and resistance aroused by what, from the medical profession's point of view, may be seen as an aggression destined to take – "rob" – from our hands the leading role in the driving of our professional activities. Such a dispute does not make sense if we don't understand once and for all the necessity to penetrate, infiltrate, understand, absorb and hybridise the border areas that contribute to nourishing, enriching and developing medical practice.

Perhaps a new Flexner Report is necessary, an indisputable diagnosis of the current state of medicine that offers precise recommendations for the changes demanded by current medical training. A meditation of this nature, carried out by a multi-disciplinary team of recognised authority could be the guide to hastening the necessary "chain reaction" that will permit the start of those changes judged to be advisable.

Medical Paradoxes could be a good departure point for understanding the problems of contemporary medicine.

I believe that in the past, and still in the present, the "heroic" novels on the great discoveries and progress of medicine, like *Microbe Hunters* by Paul de Kruif, exercised a seductive, "quasi-magic" influence on young readers. This is one of the positive influences that can be made in order to capture the best of a given generation, without which the future of our profession will enter an irretrievable limbo of unpredictable negative consequences. As already stated, the future of our noble profession depends in large part on it being capable of continuing to attract, motivate and captivate the most intellectually gifted young people to choose the study of medicine and its subsequent practice as their life's work.

THE CHALLENGES OF
CURRENT MEDICINE

The brief descriptive outline of the preceding concepts necessarily leads us to consider how to resolve potential conflicts and gain a shrewd understanding of the challenges generated by these paradoxes:

- The challenge of accepting, studying and correcting the criticism that has been made of medicine, when any support or justification is found, even when the justification often appears to be exaggerated or manipulated.
- The challenge of resolving evident contradictions in the art of practising medicine.
- The challenge of appreciating and taking advantage of the great benefits of scientific research, applying them wisely to the management of illness, without losing sight of their implicit limitations and the permanent balancing act that must occur between the technological and humanist component in medicine, where facultative behaviour must always be regulated, so that the act of medicine does not lose its true meaning.

I am optimistic about the future; man has achieved great advances and built great civilisations; science has given us an instrument of incontestable progress that enables us to correctly decipher the mysteries of nature. For that reason I share the opinion of the great American doctor, writer and thinker Lewis Thomas (1913–93) when he stated: "Epidemic disease, meteorite collisions, volcanoes, atmospheric shifts in the levels of carbon dioxide, earthquakes, excessive warming or chilling of the earth's surface are all on the worst-case list for parts of the biosphere, at one time or another, but it is unlikely that these can ever be lethal threats to a species as intelligent and resourceful as ours. We will not be wiped off the face of the earth by hard times, no matter how hard; we are tough and resilient animals, good at hard times." (Thomas, 1981)

I believe that the words "The Greatest Benefit to Mankind", the title of a book on medicine written by the British medical historian Roy Porter, represents not only everything that has been so briefly summarised here, but also the contribution that medicine has made to our species, a view that I wholly share.

REFERENCES

BOOKS

Arráiz, L. R., Uslar, P. A. 2003. *Venezuela en terapia intensive*. Venezuela: Alfadil Ediciones

Attali, J. 1981. *El orden Caníbal: Vida y muerte de la medicina*. Barcelona: Editorial Planeta (Translation from the French edition of 1979)

Beauchamp, T. L. 1987. 'Ethical Theory and the Problem of Closure'. In: Engelhardt Jr, T. H., Caplan, A. L., *Scientific Controversies, Case Studies in the Resolution and Closure of Disputes in Science and Technology*. Cambridge: Cambridge University Press

Bernard, J. 1994. *Médecin dans le siècle*. Paris: Éditions Robert Laffont

Bliss, M. 1999. *William Osler: A Life in Medicine*. Oxford: Oxford University Press

Brouwer, S. 2011. *Revolutionary Doctors: How Venezuela and Cuba Are Changing the World's Conception*. New York: NYU Press

Coleman, V. 1989. *The Health Scandal: Your Health in Crisis*. London: Mandarin Paperbacks

Cooke, R. 2001. *Dr Folkman's war: Angiogenesis and the Struggle to Defeat Cancer*. New York: Random House

Corner, G. W. 1964. *The Rockefeller Institute, 1901–1953, Origins and Growth*. New York: The Rockefeller Institute Press

Coulter, H. L., Loe Fisher, B. 1991. *A Shot in the Dark*. New York: Avery Trade

Crick, F. 1994. *The Astonishing Hypothesis: The Scientific Search for the Soul*. London: Simon & Schuster

Cushing, H. 1940. *Sir William Osler*. London: Oxford University Press

Diccionario Espasa de Medicina. 1999. Barcelona: S.L.U. Espasa Libros

Duncker, P. 1999. *James Miranda Barry*. London: Serpent's Tail

Fukuyuma, F. 2005. 'Biotechnology and the Threat of a Posthuman Future'. In: Shannon, T. A. (ed). *Genetics: Science, Ethics, and Public Policy: A Reader*. Oxford: Rowman & Littlefield Publishers

Fukuyama, F. 2002. *Our Posthuman Future: Consequences of the Biotechnology Revolution.* London: Profile Books

Fukuyuma, F. 2006. 'Our Posthuman Future'. In Winston, M & Edelbach, R. (ed). *Society, Ethics and Technology.* Boston: Wadsworth Cengage Learning

Garrett, L. 2001. *Betrayal of Trust: The collapse of global public health.* Oxford: Oxford University Press

Gawande, A. 2002. *Complications: A surgeon's notes on an imperfect science.* London: Profile Books

Gibbon, E. 1996. *The History of the Decline and Fall of the Roman Empire.* London: Penguin Classics

Gordon, R. 1993. *The Alarming History of Medicine: Amusing Anecdotes from Hippocrates to Heart Transplants.* New York: Martin's Griffin

Hamon, H. 1994. *Nos Médecins.* Paris: Éditions du Seuil

Hart, M. 1978. *The 100: A Ranking of the Most Influential Persons in History.* New York: A & W Publishers

Hart, M. 1993. *The 100: A Ranking of the Most Influential Persons in History.* Great Britain: Simon & Schuster

Hellman, H. 2001. *Great feuds in medicine: Ten of the liveliest disputes ever.* New York: John Wiley & Sons Inc.

Horton, R. 2003. *Health Wars: On the Global Frontlines of Modern Medicine.* A *New York Review* Collection

Illich, I. 1975. *Medical Nemesis: The Expropriation of Health.* London: Calder & Boyars

Illich, I. 1995. *Medical Nemesis: Limits to Medicine – The Expropriation of Health.* London: Marion Boyars Publishers

Jaén Centeno, R. 2013. *Aunque la naturaleza se opuso.* Venezuela: Cognitio

Jiménez de Asúa, L. 1928. *Libertad de amar y derecho a morir: Ensayos de un criminalista sobre eugenesia, euthanasia, endocrinología.* Madrid: Historia Nueva

Katz, J. 1984. *The Silent World of Doctor and Patient.* New York: Free Press

Kiley, R. 2001. *The Doctor's Guide to the Internet.* London: RSM

Kleinman, A. 1993. 'What is specific in western medicine?' In: Bynum, W. F., Porter, R., *Companion Encyclopedia of the History of Medicine. Vol. I.* London: Routledge

Knowles, E. (ed.) 1999. *The Oxford Dictionary of Quotations.* Oxford: Oxford University Press

Kruif de, P. 1996. *Microbe Hunters.* USA: Harcourt, Inc.

Landes, D. S. 1998. *The Wealth & Poverty of Nations: Why some are so rich and some so poor.* London: Little, Brown

Lanier, J. 2013. *Who Owns the Future?* London: Allen Lane

Le Fanu, J. 1999. *The Rise & Fall of Modern Medicine.* New York: Carroll & Graf Publishers

Le Fanu, J. 2011. *The Rise & Fall of Modern Medicine.* London: Abacus

Maddox, J. 1999. *What Remains to Be Discovered: Mapping the Secrets of the Universe, the Origins of Life, and the Future of the Human Race.* New York: Free Press

Mandelbrote, S. 2001. *Footprints of the Lion: Isaac Newton at Work.* Cambridge: Cambridge University Library

Marlatt, G. A. 1998. *Harm reduction: Pragmatic Strategies for Managing High-Risk Behaviours.* New York: The Guilford Press

Masters, R. D., McGuire, M. T. 1994. *The Neurotransmitter Revolution: Serotonin, Social Behavior, and the Law.* Carbondale: Southern Illinois University Press

McKeown, T. 1979. *The Role of Medicine: Dream, Mirage or Nemesis?* Princeton: Princeton University Press

Medawar, P. B. 1968. *The Art of the Soluble.* London: Methuen & Co. Ltd.

Mendelsohn, R. S. 1979. *Confessions of a Medical Heretic.* Chicago: Contemporary Books, Inc.

Moll, A. 2010. *Arztliche Ethik: Die Pflichten Des Arztes in Allen Beziehungen Seiner Thatigkeit* (1902). Whitefish MT, USA: Kessinger Publishing

Monro, T. K. 1951. *The Physician: As Man of Letters Science and Action.* 2nd Edition. Edinburgh: E & S. Livingstone

Murray, T. J., Bryan, C., Silverman, M. 2008. *The Quotable Osler.* Philadelphia: American College of Physicians

Nuland, S. B. 1988. *Doctors: The biography of medicine.* New York: Vintage Books

Nuland, S. B. 1997. *La sabiduría del cuerpo.* Barcelona: Grupo Editorial Norma

Nuland, S. B. 1998. *How We Live: The Wisdom of the Body*. London: Vintage

Osborne Wilson, E. 1999. *Consilience: The Unity of Knowledge*. London: Vintage

Osler, W., *c.*1892. *The Principles and Practice of Medicine: designed for the use of practitioners and students of medicine*, London: Young J. Putland

Pappworth, M. H. 1967. *Human Guinea Pigs: Experimentation on Man*. London: Routledge & Kegan Paul

Porter, R. 2001. *Bodies Politic: Disease, Death, and Doctors in Britain, 1650–1900*. Ithaca, New York: Cornell University Press

Porter, R. 2006. *Illustrated History of Medicine*, Cambridge University Press

Porter, R. 1999. *The Greatest Benefit to Mankind: A Medical History of Humanity* (The Norton History of Science). London: W. W. Norton & Company

Powell, E. 1966. In: Annas, G. J. 1998. *Some Choice: Law, Medicine, and the Market*. Oxford: Oxford University Press

Regalado de Hurtado, L., Chávez Rodríguez, C.A., 1998. *Ética e investigación: ¿el fin justifica los medios?* Peru: Pontificia Universidad Católica del Perú

Riley, J. C. 1989. *Sickness, Recovery, and Death: A History and Forecast of Ill Health*. Iowa City: University of Iowa Press

Rhodes, P. 1985. *An outline history of medicine*. London: Butterworths

de Rojas, F. 2009. *Celestina*. Sawtry: Dedalus

Saramago, J. 2013. *Blindness*, London: Vintage

Schwanitz, D. 2002. *La Cultura: Todo lo que hay que saber*. (Original title: *Bildung. Alies, was ma wissen muss*). Madrid: Antillana Ediciones Generales

Schwartz, W. B. 1998. *Life without Disease: The Pursuit of Medical Utopia*, Berkeley: University of California Press

Subramanian, V. K. 2003. *The Great Ones*. Chikhali: Abhinav Publications

Thomas, L. 1981. *Unacceptable Damage*. New York: *The New York Review of Books*

Toro Hardy, J. 1993. *Fundamentos de Teoría Económica*. Caracas: Panapo

Watts, G. 2006. 'Looking to the Future'. In: Porter, R. (ed) *The Cambridge History of Medicine*. Cambridge: Cambridge University Press

Weber, O. 1999. *French doctors*. Paris: Éditions Robert Laffont

Wilson, E. O. 1999. *Consilience: The Unity of Knowledge*. New York: Vintage

Wilson, E. O. 2002. *The Future of Life*. London: Little, Brown

Wolpert, L., Richards, A. 1998. *A Passion for Science*. Oxford: Oxford University Press

JOURNALS, REPORTS & NEWSPAPERS

Abbasi, K., Smith, R. 2003. "No More Free Lunches", *British Medical Journal*, 31 May 2003. Vol. 7400, pp.1155–6

Botbol-Baum, M. 2000. The shrinking of human rights: the controversial revision of the Helsinki Declaration. *HIV Medicine*. Volume 1, Issue 4, pp. 238–45

Statement by Betancor, J. T. (Vice President of World Federation of Right to Die Societies) 2003. In: *El País*: Madrid. 2 June 2003

Flexner, A. 1910. *Medical Education in the United States and Canada, A Report to The Carnegie Foundation for the Advancement of Teaching*. Boston: Merrymount Press.

Hogan, D. B. 1999. "Did Osler suffer from 'paranoia antitherapeuticum baltimorensis'? A comparative content analysis of The Principles and Practice of Medicine and Harrison's Principles of Internal Medicine", *CMAJ*. 11th edition. 5 October 5 1999. Vol. 161, No. 7, pp. 842–5

Jennett, B. 1985. "Intensive Care for the Elderly", *International Journal of Technology Assessment in Health Care*. January 1985. Volume. Issue 01, pp. 7–19

Medawar ,P. B. 1980. "In defense of doctors", Letter to the editor (answering Dr Thomas McKeown). *The New York Review of Books*. 15 May 1980

Osler, W. 1902. Address to the Canadian Medical Association. Montreal (17 September 1902). *The Montreal Medical Journal* Vol. XXXI. 1902

Rodgers, A. 2003. "A cure for cardiovascular disease?" *BMJ*. 26 June 2003. Vol. 326. Issue. 1407

Sackett, D. L., Rosenberg, W., Muir Gray, J. A., Haynes, R., Scott Richardson, W. 1996. Evidence based medicine: what it is and what it isn't. *BMJ*. 13 January 1996. Vol. 312. Issue 7023, pp.71–2

Smith, R. 2003. "The most important BMJ for 50 years?" *BMJ*. 28 June 2003. Vol. 326. Issue 7404

ONLINE SOURCES

Alcalá, L. E. 2006. Enfermo de pobreza, 10 January 2006. Dr. POLÍTICO (Online) (Accessed 27 August 2015) Available from: <http://doctorpolitico.com/?p=2233>

Alcalá, L. E. 2008. Ética política. 15 January 2008. Dr. POLÍTICO (Online) (Accessed 27 August 2015) Available from: <http://doctorpolitico.com/?p=2464>

Alcalá, L. E. 1986. KRISIS: Memorias Prematuras. 12 February 1986. Dr. POLÍTICO (Online) (Accessed 27 August 2015) Available from: <http://doctorpolitico.com/?p=1507>

Clínica Universidad de Navarra. 2015. *Diccionario médico: encarnizamiento terapéutico* (Online) (Accessed 6 July 2015). Available from: <http://www.cun.es/cun/diccionario-medico?letra=e&pagina=28>

Clinical Anatomy Associates. 2015. *Andreas Vesalius Bruxellensis.* (Online) (Accessed 26 June 2015) Available from: <http://clinanat.com/index.php/197-andreas-vesalius>

Collins Dictionary (Online) 2016. Paradox (Accessed 24 August 2015) Available from: <http://www.collinsdictionary.com/dictionary/english/paradox>

Encyclopædia Britannica Online 2015. R Buckminster Fuller (Accessed 24 August 2015) Available from: <http://www.britannica.com/biography/R-Buckminster-Fuller>

Feijoo, B. J. 1779. *Paradojas médicas.* (Online) (Accessed July 2015) Available from: <http://www.filosofia.org/bjf/bjft810.htm>

Hippocrates *The Hippocratic Oath.* (Online) (Accessed August 2015) Available from: <http://www.nlm.nih.gov/hmd/greek/greek_oath.html>

Jefferson, T. 1806. *President Jefferson's Letter To Dr. Edward Jenner On His Discovery of the Small Pox Vaccine, Monticello* (Online) (Accessed August 2015) Available from: <http://lachlan.bluehaze.com.au/literature.html#jefferson>

Nobelprize.org (Online) 2015. Lester Bowles Pearson – Nobel Lecture (Accessed July 2015) Available from: <http://www.nobelprize.org/nobel_prizes/peace/laureates/1957/pearson-lecture.html>

Rubin, H. 2000. *Maximum Life Span*. (Online) (Accessed August 2015)
Available from:
<www.therubins.com/aging/maximum.htm>

Today News. 2013. Cancer doctor gave needless chemo in $35M fraud,
prosecutors say. (Online) (Accessed 3 September 2015) Available from:
<www.today.com/news/cancer-doctor-gave-needless-chemo-35m-fraud-
prosecutors-say-6C10913890>

Universidad de Navarra. 2000. *Léxico de Bioética: Diagnóstico de la
muerte* (Online) (Accessed 5 July 2015) Available from:
<http://www.unav.es/cdb/dhblexico004060.html>

Universidad de Navarra. 2000. *Léxico de Bioética: Homeopatía*
(Online) (Accessed 5 July 2015) Available from:
<http://www.unav.es/cdb/dhblexico.html>

Universidad de Navarra. 2000. *Léxico de Bioética:* Órdenes de no
reanimación (Online) (Accessed 5 July 2015). Available from:
<http://www.unav.es/cdb/dhblexico.html>

Wikipedia 2015. *Encefalopatía espongiforme bovina* (Online)
(Accessed 24 August 2015) Available from:
<http://es.wikipedia.org/wiki/Encefalopat% C3%ADa_espongiforme_
bovina>

Wikipedia 2015. *Enfermedad de Creutzfeldt Jakob* (Online) (Accessed
24 August 2015) Available from:
<https://es.wikipedia.org/wiki/Enfermedad_de_Creutzfeldt-Jakob>

Wikipedia 2014. *Enfermedades de la civilización* (Online) (Accessed
25 August 2015) Available from:
<http://es.wikipedia.org/wiki/Enfermedades_de_la_civilización>

Wikipedia 2015. *Misión Barrio Adentro*. (Online) (Accessed 12 June 2015)
Available from:
<https://es.wikipedia.org/wiki/Misión_Barrio_Adentro>

Worldbank.org (Online) 2015. Health Expenditure per Capita (Accessed
July 2015) Available from:
<http://data.worldbank.org/indicator/SH.XPD.PCAP?page=2>

WIDER READING

Attali, J. 1981. *El orden Caníbal: Vida y muerte de la medicina.* Barcelona: Editorial Planeta (translation from the French edition of 1979)

Belkin, L. 1993. *First Do No Harm. The Dramatic Story of Real Doctors and Patients Making Impossible Choices at a Big-City Hospital.* New York: Ballantine Books

Bernard, C. 1957. *Introduction to the Study of Experimental Medicine,* 1865 (translated from French to English by Henry C. Greene) Boston: Transaction Publisher

Bogner, M. S. 1994. *Human Error in Medicine.* Hillsdale, N. J.: Lea

Carter, J. P. 1992. *Racketeering in medicine: The Suppression of Alternatives.* Charlottesville, VA: Hampton Road Publishing Co.

Coleman, M. L. 1991. *Cancer risk after medical treatment.* Oxford: Oxford University Press

Coles, R., Testa, R., O'Donnell, J., Armstrong, P., Brownell Anderson, M. (eds) 2003. *A Life in Medicine: A Literary Anthology.* New York: The New Press

Cooke, R. 2001. *Dr. Folkman's war: Angiogenesis and the Struggle to Defeat Cancer.* New York: Random House

D'Arcy, P. D., Griffin, J. P. 1986. *Iatrogenic diseases.* Second Edition. Oxford: Oxford University Press

Donaldson, D. 1999. *Do No Harm.* Berkley: Jove Books

Edlich, R. F., Woods, J. A., Cox, M. J. 1997. *Medicine's Deadly Dust: A Surgeon's Wake-Up Call to Society.* Clearwater, FL

Garrett, L. 2000. *Betrayal of Trust: The collapse of global public health,* New York: Hyperion

Gawande, A. 2002. *Complications: A surgeon's notes on an imperfect science.* London: Profile Books

Gendron, F. 1988. *Unexplained patient burns: investigating iatrogenic injuries.* Philadelphia: Lippincott Williams & Wilkins

Gordon, N. 2004. *Chamán.* Madrid: Ediciones B

Gordon, N. 2004. *El Médico.* Madrid: Ediciones B

Gordon, N. 2004. *La Doctora Cole.* Madrid: Ediciones B

Green, R. C. 1983. *Diseases of Medical Progress.* Philadelphia: Lippincott William & Wilkins

Green, R. C. 1983. *Medical overkill*. Philadelphia: Lippincot Williams & Wilkins

Groopman, J. 2001. *Second Opinion: Stories of Intuition and Choice in a Changing World of Medicine*. New York: Penguin Books

Hawking, S. 1998. *A Brief History of Time*. New York: Bantam Books

Hellman, H. 2001. *Great feuds in medicine: Ten of the liveliest disputes ever*. New York: John Wiley & Sons Inc.

Illich, I. 1976. *Limits to Medicine: The Expropriation of Health*, London: Marion Boyars (& Penguin 1977)

Illich, I. 1976. Medical Nemesis: *Medical Nemesis*. New York: Random House

Institute of Medicine. 2001. *Crossing the Quality Chasm: A New Health System for the 21st Century*. Washington DC: National Academic Press

Jiménez de Asúa, L. 1928. *Libertad de amar y derecho a morir: Ensayos de un criminalista sobre eugenesia, euthanasia, endocrinología*. Madrid: Historia Nueva

Katz, J. 1984. *The Silent World of Doctor and Patient*. New York: Free Press

Kohn, L. T., Corrigan, J., Donaldson, M. S. 2000. *To Err is Human: Building a Safer Health System*. Washington DC: National Academies Press

Le Fanu, J. 1999. *The Rise & Fall of Modern Medicine*. New York: Carroll & Graf Publishers

Lesueur, V. 1997. *Victimes de la médecine. Enquête sur l'erreur médicale*. Paris: Le Pré aux Clercs

Marlatt, G. A. 1998. *Harm reduction: Pragmatic Strategies for Managing High-Risk Behaviours*. New York: The Guilford Press

McKeown, T. 1979, *The Role of Medicine, Dream, Mirage or Nemesis?* Princeton NJ: Princeton University Press

Mendelsohn, R. S. 1990. *Confessions of a Medical Heretic*. New York: McGraw-Hill

Merry, A., Smith, A. M. 2001. *Errors, medicine and the law*. Cambridge: Cambridge University Press

Millenson, M. L. 1999. *Demanding medical excellence: Doctors and accountability in the information age*. Chicago: University of Chicago Press

Pappworth, M. H. 1996. *Human Guinea Pigs: Experimentation on Man*. London, Routledge & Kegan Paul

Perruca, F., Pouradier, G. 1996. *Votre santé en danger de médecine*. Paris: Michel Lafon

Reason, J. 1990. *Human Error*. Cambridge: Cambridge University Press

Robin, E. D. 1986. *Medical care can be dangerous to your health: A guide to the risks and benefits*. New York: Perrenial Library Edition

Rondberg, T. A. 1998. Under the influence of modern medicine. Chandler, AZ: *Chiropractic Journal*.

Rosenthal, M. M., Sutcliffe, K. M. (eds) 2002. *Medical error: What do we know? What do we do?* New York: John Wiley & Sons

Sánchez, S. 1996. *La médecine en flagrant délit. Le malade oublié*. Paris: Éditions de Félin

Sharpe, V. A. 1998. *Medical Harm: Historical, Conceptual and Ethical Dimensions of Iatrogenic Illness*. Cambridge: Cambridge University Press

Simms, C., Rowson, M., Marcus, R., Costello, A. 2002. *Do No Harm: Assessing the Impact of Adjustment Policies on Health*. London: Zed Books

Snedden, J. R. 2002. *Do No Harm*. St Petersburg, FL: Barclay Books LLC

Spath, P. L. 1999. *Error Reduction in Health Care: A System Approach to Improve Patient Safety*. New York: John Wiley & Sons

Weitz, M. 1982. *Health Shock: How to avoid ineffective and hazardous medical treatment*. New York: Prentice Hall

Youngson, R. M., Schott I. 1996. *Medical Blunders: Amazing True Stories of Mad, Bad, and Dangerous Doctors*. New York: New York University Press

APPENDIX

ANALYSIS OF 3RD, 5TH AND 34TH PARADOXES
Dr Augusto León C. (1918–2010)*

3rd Paradox: Vegetative life vs. Euthanasia

Essentially, the author addresses the ever-greater trend across a number of countries for the practice of assisted suicide or euthanasia as a solution for patients in a "persistent vegetative state", or for those suffering from an incapacitating painful condition.

In *Euthanasia y Suicidio Asistido* (León Cechini, 1966), I analyse the current debate at a worldwide level, the recent legislations in a number of countries, and the situation in Venezuela. I will limit myself to analysis of the latter as I am convinced that few doctors in our country are aware of the ethical and legal regulations that govern it in Venezuela.

We refer to active euthanasia (positive or direct) versus passive euthanasia (negative or indirect) (León Cechini, 1981). Active euthanasia is the deliberate act of ending a life considered to be futile, whether through suffering or for being devoid of any meaning. It is an act of commission. Death is caused through direct action or the employment of an indirect procedure. Passive euthanasia arises when a doctor ceases the use of extraordinary measures to keep a patient considered to be incurable alive, with the intention of avoiding further suffering or a persistent undefined loss of consciousness. It includes acts of omission, such as not attempting to resuscitate terminal patients or newborn

* Professor of Internal Medicine, he was President of the National Academy of Medicine in Venezuela

babies with severe congenital anomalies. Instead of postponing the end, the doctor facilitates a natural death though his or her action.

I wrote a chapter for the Venezuelan Code of Medical Ethics (Código de Deontología Médica: 1985) entitled *Del Enfermo Terminal* (Of the Terminal Patient), which falls under Title II, Chapter Four and which contains 10 Articles (71–81). I list the most significant below:

According to Article 73:

"Mentally competent patients should have the right to participate in the taking of decisions; they may refuse the use of certain diagnostic procedures; when suffering intensely they may exercise the right to seek the application of analgesics in a sufficient dosage to obtain the required relief. Likewise, they can refuse the administration of large amounts of medication if they wish to remain alert and in full consciousness of what is happening to them."

Article 77:

"The dying patient has the right to demand that they be permitted to die without the indiscriminate application of extraordinary measures to maintain life via artificial means, with respect also for their decision to not be resuscitated. Ignoring this wish can be considered a violation of the patient's right to die peacefully."

Article 80:

"Relieving human suffering is a doctor's fundamental obligation. They cannot under any circumstances deliberately cause the death of a patient if they or their family seek it."

Article 81:

"A doctor attending to an incurable patient is not obliged to use extraordinary measures to keep them alive. In these cases, where possible, the doctor will listen to the opinion of other medical professionals. The doctor will follow whatever may be written in the Medical Practice Law Regulations."

In conclusion, between us according to Articles 73, 77 and 81 of the Venezuelan Code of Medical Ethics, the practice of passive euthanasia is permissible. Active euthanasia is banned, as stated in Article 80 of the quoted Code. Whilst it does not refer to terminal patients, the content of Article 69 included in the Chapter entitled *De los Derechos y Deberes de los Enfermos* (Of the Rights and Duties of Patients – Title II, Chapter Three) can be considered as supplementary to the articles quoted. It says the following: "A mentally competent adult patient has the right to refuse certain diagnostic and therapeutic indications. The right to self-determination cannot be rescinded by society unless the practice of the same interferes with the rights of others."

In Venezuela the practice of assisted suicide violates the ethical and legal regulations set out in Articles 80 of the Code of Medical Ethics and 414 of the Venezuelan Penal Code (Código Penal Venezolano, 1964) respectively, of which the latter is transcribed here: "He who induces any individual to commit suicide or in any way helps them will be punished, if the suicide occurs, with a sentence of seven to ten years."

REFERENCES
1   León-Cechini, A. 1966. *Eutanasia y Suicidio Asistido.* Caracas, Venezuela. Rev Fed Med Venez. 4 (2): 115–122.
2   León-Cechini, A. 1981. *Eutanasia. Trabajo de Incorporación como Individuo de Número para ocupar el Sillón IX de la Academia Nacional de Medicina.* Caracas: Ediciones AMON, C. A.
3   *Código de Deontología* Médica. Aprobado durante la LXXVI Reunión Extraordinaria de la Asamblea de la Federación Médica Venezolana realizada en Caracas. 29/03/85.
4   *Código Penal Venezolano.* Gaceta Oficial No 915 del 30/06/64.

5th Paradox: Lies vs. State secrets

Should the public be kept informed of the health of their leaders?

We live in a time in which public figures, dead or alive, are the subject of biographies written by their private doctors, friends, writers or journalists in general.

The publication in life or posthumously of details of the health problems of known statesmen and heads of state poses a very delicate question about whether doctors have the right to divulge confidential information about their patients, with many maintaining the right to tell without it constituting a violation of the general rule of upholding professional secrecy. Some believe that we are obliged to satisfy the public's morbid desire to know the details of notable figures' illnesses and the final words uttered from their deathbeds, on the condition that this disclosure does not discredit, but rather contributes to a greater understanding of the person thereby enhancing their reputation.

It is also said that the doctor is not just the "patient's doctor", but that they also play a public role in bringing tranquillity to the population with regards to everything concerning the state of their leaders' health. Therefore, under certain circumstances there is justification for an exception to the rule that health is a matter more private than of public peace; and if in life no information whatsoever should be revealed without the consent of the patient, after their death it is appropriate to do so in order for "the lessons of history to permit an evaluation of similar situations that will inevitably be repeated".

In Chapter 36 of *Ética en Medicina* (León-Cechini, 1973) I dedicate a section (*Preguntas y Respuestas*) to the issue in hand, with analyses of the illness and death of Simón Bolívar, Lord Moran's biography with regards to the illness of his patient Winston Churchill, the illness and death of Franklin Delano Roosevelt, John F. Kennedy's adrenal glands, Eisenhower's regional enteritis.

I believe that we should distinguish between two entirely different situations:

1. Regardless of how important the patient is, medical information should not be revealed in their lifetime without their prior consent. The doctor-patient privilege is enshrined in law in order to prevent the legal use of information supplied by the patient against them under certain circumstances. Aside from being a matter of ethics and good taste, as well as being a legal right, confidence is a patient's basic right by which their private life is respected; and this privilege should not clash with the doctor's right to divulge information demanded by the public, unless said doctor is prepared to become a media puppet.

2. Something wholly different, although no less debatable is the possibility of divulging confidences posthumously in the interests of the State and community in general. For example, the right of Venezuelans and citizens of other countries to know the details of the illness and death of the Liberator (Simón Bolívar) is acceptable; the same could be said of other great figures in history. If it is necessary, the disclosure of this information must be done at the right time, with respect for the truth, without lurid details and without damaging their reputation, as "If illness, as man's most vulnerable state leads to greater knowledge, the precision and purity of the description should be parallel to its higher objectives." (Conde-Jahn, 1963)

3. We cannot let this opportunity pass without referring to the unscrupulous doctor, who acts like a hack by trade and takes advantage of their position as private doctor to an important person by divulging intimacies about them in life or death with the grim intention of elevating their own prestige or making themselves known to the public through very un-decent means.

Chapter VI of Title I of the Venezuelan Law of Medical Practice, which discusses medical secrets, does not consider the situations we have just analysed. Instead, Article 132 of the *Código de Deontología Médica* (Venezuelan Code of Medical Ethics, 1985) provides valuable information in the section entitled Professional Secrets (Chapter I of Title IV). It is transcribed here:

> Article 132: The doctor must respect the secrets confided to them or those of which they are made aware during their professional conduct, even after the death of the patient.
>
> However much time has passed after death, this duty does not diminish as there is no time limit in this respect, and the disclosure of certain facts could damage not only the memory and good name of the deceased, but also their family.
>
> Sole paragraph: The possibility of communicating a confidence in the interests of the State and community in general after the death of the patient is a different matter. In the case of it being necessary, the disclosure of this information must be done at the right time, with respect for the truth, without entering into lurid details and without damaging the deceased's reputation. The precision and purity of the description should be parallel to its higher objectives.

REFERENCES
1   León-Cechini, A. 1973. *Ética en Medicina.* Barcelona, Madrid, Rio de Janeiro, México: Editorial Científico – Médica
2   Conde-Jahn, F. 1963. Discurso pronunciado en la apertura de la sesión preliminar histórico-científica sobre la enfermedad y muerte del Libertador. In: *Enfermedad y Muerte del Libertador.* Caracas: Lit. y Tip. Vargas
3   *Código de Deontología* Médica, 29-03-85, Caracas, Venezuela

34th Paradox: The truth vs. The partial truth

In the work *La Muerte y el Morir* (León-Cechini, 1980), I dedicate an extensive chapter to *La Verdad y el Enfermo* (Truth and the Patient). A section of the same work addresses the issue of *La Verdad y el Enfermo Terminal* (Truth and the Terminal Patient). I have extracted the following commentaries from two other publications of mine. (León-Cechini, 1982 & 1993)

According to the experience of numerous authors, practically all patients suffering from a malignant disease "know" in one way or another the severity of the disease they are suffering from. What is appropriate is to try to understand how the patient is dealing with it privately, how they are facing up to the menace, the mechanisms they have developed to conceal it and how we can be of assistance.

What upsets, sometimes horrifies, these patients to a greater degree is not the fear that they are going to die, but a growing fear of loneliness, a feeling of abandonment. And it is precisely this that the doctor can help to dispel.

There are three arguments presented by those who justify lying to the patient: protecting them because they would not understand, because they really don't want to know the truth, or because knowledge of their illness could damage them.

The situation needs to be analysed from another perspective. Lying is contrary to the patient's right to know the truth about something that concerns them more than anybody else, not to mention the psychological and practical benefits that stem from being able to avoid the unnecessary and damaging treatments they could be subjected to if the real condition is ignored. There are few patients who clearly demand not to be informed if they think it is bad news. Others may not say it, but do give clear signs of their vulnerability when faced with the potential anguish.

The issue resides with we the doctors: we have to learn to confront patients' problems; we have to learn the language and attitudes required to speak to them about their difficulties. We have to train ourselves to know how to bring up the options and, what's more, dare to consider the following possibility: what would I want for myself or for my loved ones in the same situation?

The dilemma for patients resides in knowing if they can believe their doctors, in knowing if their wishes will be respected. The majority of doctors who decide that their patients don't really want to know the truth are scared of the truth themselves, only an intelligent and humane doctor will manage to suppress or ease this suffering.

Let us carefully consider the following three statements:

1. The capacity to understand what a patient wants or can tolerate does not require scientific judgement
2. Lying to a patient is not permissible, however, holding back the truth until the right moment is different to lying
3. If it is morally unacceptable to lie, telling the truth therefore becomes a moral obligation, however, the duty to not lie is not equivalent to the duty to always tell the truth.

The patient has the right to know the truth and it is the doctor's duty to reveal it. But it is also true that the patient has other rights and one of them is "the right to not know". Indeed, they can indirectly indicate their desire to ignore the truth or explicitly indicate it. In these circumstances, does the doctor have the right to invoke their obligation to not disrespect the truth, and interfere with the patient's wishes?

For some doctors the truth is an obsession that leads them to the extreme situation of transforming said obligation into an act more of cruelty than of real honesty, where any humanitarian consideration is put to one side.

"What I would like, doctor, is the complete truth." Over long years of professional practice, doctors have learned, sometimes painfully, that this complete truth is often the last thing that the patient wishes to know, and that the intensity of their demands is in inversely proportional relation to the real desire of being provided with the information with which such vehemence they feign to demand.

The white lie, lying by necessity, poses a difficult problem for moral philosophers. For them veracity as a value, with its specific moral weight, does not permit exceptions: the necessary lie would be an anti-value, at least from the point of view of veracity as an absolute value.

We the doctors find ourselves obliged to handle it from different perspectives. In certain circumstances we are faced with serious moral problems; situations before which there remains no other alternative than to lie, due to the collision of our obligation to the truth and an even higher value for us: human suffering. What justifies and values certain decisions is genuine moral intention, which inevitably drives us to decide on one value over another. Between the duty to the truth and the duty to help the patient there can be no conflict of interests. A doctor who avoids making decisions, who remains neutral, violates both values and shows intolerable cowardice.

For those who consider that it is always incorrect to deliberately lie to the patient in benefit of the latter, I would answer that it is also incorrect to tell them the truth at the least appropriate time. Eliminating all residue of hope is inhumane. The truth, or rather what we honestly believe to be the truth, expressed in the appropriate way and at the right moment is in certain situations the only way to combat the anxiety and uncertainty felt by a patient facing the unknown.

REFERENCES

1 León-Cechini, A. 1980. *La Muerte y el Morir.* Caracas: Cromotip
2 León-Cechini, A. 1982. *¿Dónde se halla la verdad?* Caracas: Tribuna Médica
3 León-Cechini, A. 1993. *La Verdad, el Médico y el Enfermo. Ciencia al Día.* No. 3

ANALYSIS OF PARADOXES 6, 16 AND 17
Dr J. M. Avilán Rovira

6th Paradox: Consuming alcohol vs. Good health

Studies continue on the effect of alcohol on health. The results of a study carried out by a group studying the aetiology and natural history of atherosclerosis in communities were published in January 2004 (the "Atherosclerosis Risk in Communities Study", better known by its initials: ARIC). (Ding et al, 2004)

Of a total of almost 16,000 patients studied, with ages ranging between 45 and 64 and resident in various American communities, just over 2,800 patients of 55 years old or older were selected at random to undertake a brain magnetic resonance imaging scan (MRI). After excluding those who provided no information on alcohol consumption in any way, they examined 1,935 people, distributed in approximate proportions according to gender and race. The basic characteristics of those not eligible or who declined to participate in the test were similar to those submitted to the MRI.

The objective was to evaluate the association between alcohol consumption and cerebral abnormalities detected by the MRI, with the aim of understanding the effect that moderate and low alcohol consumption has on the brain. As we are aware, few known studies have examined this association in population groups.

An MRI permits the direct observation of structural changes in the brain, and previous studies have demonstrated that cerebral infarction and white matter lesions can predict strokes. Likewise, it is accepted that cerebral atrophy is associated with cognitive poverty and reduction of motor function.

Statistical analyses to evaluate the association between cerebral lesions and the consumption of alcohol are carried out prior to the adjustment of demographic factors (age, gender, race), BMI, smoking habits, income, exercise and diabetes.

In contrast with the results of a study on cardiovascular health (Mukamal et al, 2001), no protective link was found between medium or low alcohol consumption and cerebral infarction. However, in correspondence with the aforementioned study, a positive association was found between the consumption of alcohol and cerebral atrophy.

This relationship between alcohol consumption and cerebral atrophy was consistent both in men and women, white or black, and in dose-response function.

The explanatory mechanism of the link between the two is still not clear. Alcohol can directly contribute to atrophy with an adverse effect on neurons and their components, or even indirectly, through hyper-tension or heat arrhythmias that reduce the flow of blood to the brain, for example. The authors cite studies that have established that cerebral atrophy and neurological deficiencies related to or induced by chronic alcohol abuse can be partially reversed via sustained abstinence. (Pfefferbaum et al, 1995 & Sullivan et al, 2000)

The results of these studies and those that will surely follow will contribute new elements, facilitating further discussion of this paradox.

REFERENCES

1   Ding J., Eigenbrodt M.L., Mosley T. H., Jr, Hutchinson R.G., Folsom A.R., Harris T. B., et al. 2004. Alcohol intake and cerebral abnormalities on magnetic resonance imaging in a community-based population of middle-aged

adults: the Atherosclerosis Risk in Communities (ARIC) study. *Stroke.* 35 (1): 16–21

2   Mukamal K. J., Longstreth W. T. Jr, Mittleman M. A., Crum R.M., Siscovick D. S. 2001. Alcohol consumption and subclinical findings on magnetic resonance imaging of the brain in older adults: The Cardiovascular Health Study. *Stroke.* 32 (9): 1939–1946

3   Pfefferbaum A., Sullivan E. V., Mathalon D. H., Shear P. K., Rosenbloom M. J., Lim K. O. 1995. Longitudinal changes in magnetic resonance imaging brain volumes in abstinent and relapsed alcoholics. *Alcohol Clin Exp Res.* 19 (5): 1177-1191.

4   Sullivan E. V., Rosenbloom M. J., Lim K. O., Pfefferbaum A. 2000. Longitudinal changes in cognition, gait, and balance in abstinent and relapsed alcoholic men: Relationships to changes in brain structure. *Neuropsychology.* 14 (2): 178 – 188.

16th Paradox: Clinic vs. Laboratory

It is interesting to note that in a little-known work by Doctor Luis Razetti, entitled *Sobre las relaciones que deben existir entre el laboratorio y la clínica* (On the relationship that should exist between laboratory and clinic), given on 25 December 1906 at the Vargas Society of Medicine Students, the great wise man of that time drew attention to the powerful force of attraction that the laboratory had on young students, to the detriment of the hospital.

In December 1929, 23 years after he gave the conference, he wrote an "addition", as he called it, in the *Gaceta Médica de Caracas* (Razetti, 1929) where he said that his opinions remained the same with regard to the relationship that exists between the laboratory and the clinic.

The message for students at the beginning of the century, and later for readers of the *Gaceta*, was "it is not the laboratory men who make the diagnosis, nor they who prescribe treatments; it is we the doctors who interpret the laboratory data, and, having questioned and examined the patient, establish a firm diagnosis of the illness."

It is surprising that the book *Clinical Epidemiology,* (Sackett et al, 1991) which was published some fifty-six years later, states "diagnostic data go far beyond those that are generated in the clinical chemistry laboratory, the radiology department, or the pathology service . . . the clinical data obtained by taking a thoughtful history and performing a purposeful physical examination are far more powerful than anything obtained in the diagnostic laboratory and are usually quite sufficient to establish a definitive diagnosis". (Sackett et al, 1991: p.51)

One of the problems with diagnostic test results is the interpretation of "normalcy", for which there are up to six definitions. (Sackett et al, 1991: pp.58–59) The limits of "normal" in the majority of diagnostic tests are determined by assessments carried out on a large number of subjects and arbitrarily defined as the range between two standard deviations on each side of the arithmetical average. In laboratory results, these are known as "normal values". Many doctors are unaware that of those tested, one in twenty patients will present results beyond or below the "normal range", without being unwell. This probability increases as more independent tests are carried out. So for example, an "SMA-20" can reach 64%. (Black, 2002: p.14) The lack of awareness of this fact can lead to unnecessary additional studies or potentially dangerous treatments.

A number of studies have demonstrated the factors that can influence diagnostic test results, independently of the illness, such as age, sex, body position at the time of taking the specimen, time of the day, tourniquet pressure, length of time processing the specimen, etc. (Black, 2002: pp. 13–14) An aspect that is generally neglected is the reliability and reproducibility of the results. Concordance of intra-observer and inter-observer variability is the point at which we the doctors start evaluating the results, assessing the obviously subjective work of radiologists, histopathologists, cytopathologists, and even the less obviously subjective laboratory observations, such as flocculation, dark fields, and white blood cell differential counts. (Feinstein, 2002: p.448)

Clinical Diagnosis and the Laboratory, published in 1986 by Year Book Medical Publishers, was intended to help doctors interpret the results of diagnostic tests. However, due to the fact that it only covered 40 diagnostic problems the first edition of *Diagnostic Strategies for Common Medical Problems* was circulated in 1991, with a second broadened and updated edition appearing in 1999.

In 1946, the year I graduated, the slogan was "the diagnosis is suspected by the doctor and confirmed by the laboratory". At that time, however, diagnostic test results, including laboratory tests, were interpreted as they currently are with tests known as criterion or gold standard. Thus, if the results were positive or abnormal, they would confirm the suspected illness. If negative or normal, they would discount the illness.

It was not until 1947 that a group of doctors working with epidemiologist Jacob Yerushalmy registered observer variability and conformity indices in X-Ray procedures. In that same year, Yerushalmy introduced the terms sensitivity and specificity, which are still the established indices for interpreting diagnostic test results today. (Yerushalmy: 1947)

REFERENCES

1   Razetti L. 1929. Relaciones que deben existir entre el laboratorio y la clínica. *Gac Méd Caracas.* 36 (24): 341–346
2   Sackett D. L., Brian Haynes R., Guyatt, G., Tugwell P. 1991. *Clinical Epidemiology: A Basic Science for Clinical Medicine.* Second Edition. Boston: Little, Brown & Co
3   Black E. R., Bordley D. R., Tape G. T., Panzer R. J. 1991. *Diagnostic strategies for common medical problems.* Philadelphia. American College of Physicians
4   Feinstein A. R. 2002. *Principles of Medical Statistics.* Boca Raton: Chapman & Hall

5   Yerushalmy J. 1947. Statistical problems in assessing methods of medical diagnosis, with special reference to X-ray techniques. *Public Health Rep.* 62 (40): 1432–1449

17th Paradox: Essential examinations vs. Optional examinations

The University of Ontario publication *Clinical Epidemiology* examines and evaluates diagnostic strategies, including the "exhaustion strategy". (Sackett et al, 1991: pp.10–13) According to the authors this is carried out in two stages. First, all possible relevant data is collected. Only once this is achieved does the search for a diagnosis through this data mountain begin. That is, a data bank is created and then a diagnosis is considered. This procedure results in numerous unnecessary and costly assessments, as well as going against a scientific approach.

In that regard, the authors cite the results of an investigation carried out in 1976 in Adelaide, Australia and published by Timothy Durbridge and colleagues in the Medical Journal of Australia. (cited in Sackett et al, 1991 p.14) The authors randomly divided 1,500 patient admissions into two groups: one group underwent a series of 50 tests and the other didn't. This exhaustive search, prior to any clinical examination or background, did not produce any decrease in mortality, morbidity, duration of monitoring, disability, medical opinions on patient development, or length of hospitalisation. The admission screening only produced an increase in the cost of care and a decline in patient satisfaction.

These days, the theory and practice of interpreting diagnostic tests is included in the training of future doctors, with the aim of streamlining the diagnostic process and achieving a medical practice that is more scientific, more human and more in tune with moral codes.

This is why the concept of traits and characteristics in diagnostic tests, such as sensitivity and specificity (which are starting to be substituted by more operative concepts like likelihood ratios) are the domain of our undergraduate doctors, postgraduate residents and clinical professors in the main national university hospitals.

However, nearly twenty years' experience in postgraduate internal medicine at the University Hospital in Caracas permits my summary of the application of this knowledge to practical medicine, as set out below.

The diagnosis process requires two essential steps. The first is the establishment of hypothetical or possible diagnoses, followed by an attempt to reduce the number of potential diagnoses by progressively discounting specific diseases. This process requires very sensitive tests, or high sensitivity tests as is often said. The next step is the search for the diagnosis of highest clinical suspicion. This process requires a very specific test, or a high specificity test. Essentially, when the results are abnormal this test should confirm the presence of the disease.

Up until this point, the words of Griner in his very well-known work have practically been repeated word for word. (Griner et al, 1981)

Nevertheless, one of the warnings stated in this same work and again in Black et al (1999) (to which nobody appears to pay any attention, is that "a diagnostic test cannot be interpreted properly without considering what the probability of disease was before the diagnostic test of procedure result was obtained." (Griner et al, 1999: p.18)

If we understand diagnosis as a process of investigation whereby a hypothesis is suggested, accepted or refuted according to collected data, incorporating the previous probability is an indispensible step, as without this it is impossible to interpret the results of the ordered diagnostic tests (and therefore use them rationally).

Without an a priori probability (the estimate made prior to the diagnostic test results), it isn't possible to estimate the posterior probability, that is to say the probability that our patient has the suspected disease if the result of the test is positive, or by contrast does not have the disease if the result is negative.

278

How are a priori or pre-test probabilities estimated? Many people are reluctant to attempt an estimate for which not even general rules exist, especially given that the estimate would lead to a personal, subjective quantification, a piece of data classified as "soft", as it is scornfully described in professional slang, as opposed to valid and reliable "hard" data.

However, it is necessary to keep in mind that it isn't possible to interpret diagnostic test results without this background clinical information, unless it is perfect, that is to say one hundred per cent sensitive, one hundred per cent specific, which is very rare.

One of the indispensible requirements for obtaining this background clinical information is through approaching the client, or as Otto Lima Gómez says, "stopping at the patient's side", with the earnest intention of helping them, literally and essentially fulfilling the doctor's primary role to attend, help, *adsistere*, or stop at another's side. (Lima-Gómez, 1999)

It is through the taking of a patient's history and physical examination (with these being understood as the gathering of a group of diagnostic tests, not mere routine tests) and through knowledge not only of the current illness, but also of its history and possible origins, that we learn to estimate the likelihood, the prior probability, that the patient is suffering from the illness we suspect. It is true that this a priori probability before tests will be subjective (given that it is assessed by the doctor), but the more the probability is based in objective "hard" data achieved through questioning and a physical examination guided by the patient's complaints, the more valid it will be.

Thus, in order to develop the probability of an illness before ordering tests, we need to combine what we may know about the prevalence of the illness, the patient risk factors for the condition and the rate at which the pattern of symptoms and signs manifested by the patient concur with the pattern of the suspected illness. (Black et al, 1999: p.19)

We cannot expand on this any further, but believe we have drawn attention once more to the importance of a priori or pre-test probability estimates in correctly interpreting diagnostic tests. A command of this knowledge is essential for the rational ordering of the required tests, in order to avoid wasting time and money in the search for the well-being that they deserve, that is to say, diminishing elective assessments and making a more professional selection of essential examinations.

The references cited below are recommended:

REFERENCES

1   Sackett D. L., Brian Haynes R., Guyatt, G., Tugwell P. 1991. *Clinical Epidemiology: A Basic Science for Clinical Medicine*. Second Edition. Boston: Little Brown & Co.

2   Griner F. P., Mayewski R. J., Mushlin A. I., Greenland Ph. 1981. *Selection and interpretation of diagnostic tests and procedures*. Ann Int Med. 94 (4 – Part 2): 553– 600

3   Lima-Gómez O. 1999. *Vigencia de la aproximación clínica al paciente. Análisis de dos mil historias clínicas*. Gaceta Médica Caracas. 107 (2) 204–208

4   Black E. R., Bordley D. R., Tape G. T., Panzer R. J. 1991. *Diagnostic strategies for common medical problems*. Philadelphia. American College of Physicians

ADDENDUM

I want to express my deep gratitude to Luis Enrique Alcalá, Elías Anzola Pérez, Antonio Clemente H, Eduardo Colmenares Finol, Jorge Díaz Polanco, Alejandro Goic Goic, Mauricio Goihman, Rubén Jaén Centeno, Ernesto Kahan, Francisco A. Kerdel, Martha Ramos de Kerdel, Luisa Sofía Kerdel de Blatnik, Aníbal J. Latuff, Eduardo Mathison, Rafael Muci Mendoza (who offered me the additional honour of writing the prologue to this book), Karem Noris-Suárez, José Félix Oletta, José Félix Patiño, Rubén Darío Peralta, Jaime Piquero, Pablo A. Pulido, Arturo Ramos Caldera, Eduardo J. Santaella, Raúl Sanz Machado and Gustavo Vollmer, who read the manuscript of the book and corrected any errors of spelling or syntax. If any errors remain they are my sole responsibility. When at my invitation these readers first contributed their comments on the content of the text, I thought it important, necessary even, to incorporate them as an addendum to the book, which I do here.

EDUARDO COLMENARES FINOL

I have read *Medical Paradoxes* and can declare that it is not only of great interest for doctors and students of medicine, but also for the general public, amongst which I include myself.

These paradoxes, written as they are in simple language, are such interesting and fascinating narratives that they have helped me to reflect on a number of political issues.

I include below a few notes on those paradoxes deserving of particular comment:

1st Paradox: The science of medicine vs. The art of medicine

The debate on how much art or science exist in subjects as "scientific" as medicine and engineering is really very interesting. According to the dictionary one definition of art that could be closest to this paradox is: "set of precepts and rules necessary to do a job well". In that respect, good doctors are those who practise "art" well in medical science, which when viewed from this perspective appears to coincide with what Medawar expressed. However, I was drawn to the increasingly frequent appearance of the "technologist doctor" (Paradox 46) who is not very scientific, who uses computer diagnostic programmes, who feeds the machine with symptoms, only for the diagnosis and the treatment to be produced by the printer and signed off by the "doctor".

2nd Paradox: Demographic explosion vs. Quality of life

This is a fascinating topic. As you say: "will medicine become a victim of its own success?" If we study history we find that as well as illness and epidemics, wars used to be another indirect way of controlling demographic growth. We could therefore conclude: will peace also be a victim of its own success? The answer is obvious: not even times of peace or medical advancement have anything to do with the consequences of humanitarian intentions. The solution to that enigma has to be answered by the political class who need to face up to these problems. Will world leaders confront that problem in peace and not in war? I hope that they will, even when the difficulty lies in the fact that those people who reproduce the most are the less educated, so whilst they may be in the minority today, they will eventually come to be the majority and therefore modern demographics could lead to political power belonging to the ignorant.

282

8th Paradox: Staying in one's country of origin vs. Emigration

Apart from political and economic causes, as mentioned, there is another reason that is linked to globalisation. These days, employment markets for well-trained professionals like doctors and engineers are global. For example, in Abu Dhabi one will find German, Australian, Italian etc. doctors in well-paid jobs, who have chosen to save hard currency and then return to their countries with funds that would have taken much longer to obtain in their country of origin.

14th Paradox: Employees vs. Administrators

Medicine and engineering are increasingly more complex; they have gone from being the practice of liberal professionals to a teamwork exercise, in which the red tape of managerial coordination intervenes. Unfortunately, management skills don't appear to be a very desirable attribute for university-trained doctors. This leads me to mention a very relevant fact for our country. It is very difficult to imagine a Ministry of Health with a minister who is not a doctor, and the same applies to the president of the Venezuelan Institute of Social Security. This point leads me to relay the case of my sister-in-law, who is a nurse, a graduate of the University of Georgetown and who began her career in the Washington DC public hospital system. After obtaining a master's degree in Hospital Administration from the same university, she became on her own merit the leading authority in the Public Health System of Washington DC, where an average of 50,000 people were attended to each day. Of course, there are doctors, like my brother-in-law, who are as good a doctor as they are a manager.

15th Paradox: The medical act: Complete vs. Partial

I have a life story that touches on this very important issue and is reflected in Paradox 26: *Humility vs. Arrogance and dogma*. One night, at the age of 30, whilst giving classes at the Central University of

Venezuela, I had a nervous breakdown (mental exhaustion). My wife spoke to my brother-in-law and he referred me to a cardiologist at the Ávila Clinic. The cardiologist didn't find anything cardiovascular and referred me to an internist at the same clinic, and as this person didn't find anything either, I was referred to a psychiatrist. I had follow up appointments with each of the three doctors, and when I attended the appointments I realise that they had each prescribed me the same medication in three different dosages. I mistakenly thought that treatment for my illness was being coordinated by one of the doctors. Eventually, I went to see my uncle, who at the time was Head of Medical Services at the Military Hospital. After a series of examinations he concluded that in addition to the "nervous breakdown", I had contracted another illness caused by the very same doctors I had seen. He gave it the name iatrogenesis, which is featured in Paradox 35.

22nd Paradox: Politicians vs. The medical profession

I think you are right to criticise the excesses of political improvisation, such as "guaranteeing health". But ultimately I agree with Virchow that there is a close relationship between medicine and well-meaning politics, in so far as they are each seeking welfare.

But equally, as one has to distinguish between good and bad doctors or empirical healers in medicine, politics is also full of improvisers and empiricists. It is the only science, in our medium, that confuses political science with law.

33rd Paradox: Local medicine vs. Global medicine

I like the metaphor "ocean of oil". Globalisation is an ocean of oil in which a country either learns to sail, or straggles behind and drowns.

47th Paradox: Medical progress vs. Socio-economic progress

It is correct that all progress needs a culture to interpret, understand and accept it. The same occurs in politics; progress is only achieved in an

284

environment of political culture, and culture is a generational matter that only becomes established over time.

59th Paradox: Biomedical research: Duty of the State vs. Philanthropic institutions' contribution

The work coordinated between the State and the private sector is essential, as much for health as for education. This leads me to Soviet Marxist propaganda, it was often said that the Soviet health systems were free and of excellent quality when this couldn't have been further from the truth. My daughter was in the USSR for nearly a year at the beginning of the nineties, and recounts how a Venezuelan friend became unwell and was admitted to a Moscow hospital; she left terrified of the service and the quality of the doctors.

ALEJANDRO GOIC GOIC

I think the book is excellent. It addresses very completely the most relevant issues and uncertainties faced by contemporary medicine, as much from the point of view of care for the individual as that of the organisation of a population's healthcare, in its delicate medical, social, cultural, economical, and political corners. Identifying one hundred paradoxes in medicine is no small matter: the comprehensiveness of your essay and your broad medical experience speak to us. The opinions expressed on each of the subjects are to me very appropriate and pertinent. The book is based on solid documentation, and offers relevant information and varied and valuable historical records, it is easy to read and, moreover, entertaining.

The book contains issues that are essential to highlight in our time in order to motivate consideration of the complex problem of medical care and public health by doctors, students of medicine, political leaders and the enlightened public. Yet your optimistic vision of the future is stimulating and encouraging.

RÚBÉN JAÉN CENTENO

The author of this work possesses an exceptional wealth of knowledge, which he communicates to us simply, and which could enormously benefit an increase in the culture of doctors and people interested in knowing the facts beyond those presented as immutable truths. I believe this to be a very useful reference book. Those who memorise its content will have an enviable general knowledge.

ERNESTO KAHAN

Analysis of 68th Paradox: Curative medicine vs. Preventative medicine
Effectively, as Dr Francisco Kerdel-Vegas states: "These are not actually opposing or contradictory actions, in fact they are complementary." In the past we were accustomed to differentiating between activities called promotion of health, prevention and curing. Promotion was the great chapter of health education, prevention was principally related to vaccinations, and finally curing was related to the therapeutic measures intended to repair health affected by diseases.

The implementation and generalised use of diagnostic methods in a seemingly healthy population was intended to detect hidden disease processes so that early and effective treatment could begin, it has also enabled us to distinguish between three different stages or levels of prevention: Primary, secondary and tertiary prevention. On the one hand, this level of differentiation permitted the unification of the afore-mentioned complementary activities into one sole process dependent

286

on the natural history of the disease; it also had the objective of achieving a modified history of the disease.

The following illustration, adapted from the book *Clinical Epidemiology, The Essentials* (Fletcher *et al*, 1991: 155–70), demonstrates the focus of attention and limitations of the three aforementioned levels of prevention, within the context of the natural history of the disease.

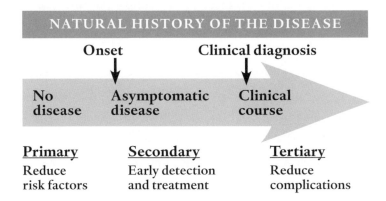

In diseases that have not yet begun, such as poliomyelitis, lung cancer or AIDS, action needs to be taken in order to stop the disease from occurring; risk factors need to be removed or infection should be avoided through vaccines. In the aforementioned examples this means being inoculated against poliomyelitis, not smoking to avoid lung cancer, using contraception and avoiding promiscuous sexual relations with regards to AIDS.

When the illness is still unapparent but in an incubation period or clinically silent, the objective of prevention is to screen those illnesses where diagnostic means and effective treatments exist in order to achieve early detection of the corresponding disease, and in those subjects seemingly exposed to the risks of becoming unwell, the objective is to identify them and establish a specific existing treatment.

This process of examining seemingly healthy individuals is not perfect and has levels of sensitivity (capacity for capturing truly positive cases of the illness) and specificity (capacity for rejecting untrue cases of the illness), which are gauged by percentage and evidence.

When the disease is in clinical course, generally chronic illnesses, tertiary prevention is important through application of methods or treatments so that complications of all type and level can be avoided, with death being the most serious. Two examples are the treatment of diabetes with antihyperglycaemic drugs, and the treatment of cardiac arrhythmia with anticoagulants.

With these prevention processes there are ethical problems at all levels, from informing the patient and their relatives, financial aspects that influence prioritisation, evaluation of contraindications, reliability of procedures based on "clinical evidence", and legalities.

In a study carried out in Israel, we demonstrate that the majority of cases of urinary tract infections (the most common urinary infection in women) were not treated according to current treatment guidelines. Non-recommended and costly antibiotics were used instead. These results indicate the necessity for the implementation of medical education programmes on this issue within the health care system. (Kahan et al. 2003)

In another study we demonstrate that there are breaches in many areas of cancer detection programmes due to factors related to the doctor, to the patient's education, to the specific allocation of funds for health services, to the distribution of guidelines, and to the population's access to corresponding services. (Kahan & El-Najjar. 2007)

REFERENCES

1   Fletcher R. H., Fletcher S. W., Wagner E. H. 1991. *Epidemiology: A Basic Science for Clinical Medicine*. Second Edition. Boston: Little, Brown & Co.
2   Kahan E., Kahan N., Chinitz D. P. 2003. *Urinary Tract Infection in Women: Physician's Preferences for Treatment and Adherence to Guidelines:*

A National Drug Utilization Study in a Managed Care Setting. European Journal of Clinical Pharmacology; 59 (8–9): 663–668

3   Kahan E., K El-Najjar. 2007. *Primary care physicians' perceived barriers to cancer prevention and control. Comparison in two different environments.* Archivos en Medicina Familiar. 9 (1) 49-60 (In English with abstract in Spanish)

Analysis of 89th Paradox: Family medicine vs. Community medicine

Dr Francisco Kerdel-Vegas, author of this important book, opens this paradox, this dilemma even, with great clarity, with the concept of continuity in medical care as a characteristic of the family medicine specialism. "The name family medicine indicates an integral primary care system. In family medicine the doctor does not just see the patient for an initial consultation, but will also follow through any possible procedures by medical specialists, remaining responsible for their patient throughout."

The conceptual essence of this relatively new idea in medical attention cannot be understood without this continuity and other guidelines, which I will attempt to analyse here in the most succinct way possible. However, in my understanding it is no different to the old approach of the "family doctor", as my father was accustomed to define himself when we practised our profession in a remote town in Argentine Patagonia in the first half of the twentieth century.

The World Organization of Family Doctors (WONCA) was officially founded in Melbourne in 1972 (Organización Mundial de Médicos de Familia, 1996), amid many declarations and recommendations. At its congress in November 1994 it established that medical practice should ideally be personalised, health-oriented and community-based, that every person should know their family doctor and be personally known by them, that the family doctor should be well-trained (WONCA lobbies for this), able to provide adequate answers for the majority of health problems presented communally by the greater part of the public, and that all countries should provide postgraduate training specifically in family medicine. (*La contribución del médico de familia.* 1996)

In fact, the birth and subsequent development of family medicine was directly preceded by Community-Oriented Primary Care (COPC), and provides a conceptual foundation for the involved educators and practising doctors. (Longlett et al., 2001) COPC, which is universally defended due to its initial success in the 1950s, continues to be hard for primary medical care doctors and educators to interpret, thereby making its implementation awkward. (Kahan, 2007)

One of the countries in which the concept of the family doctor has developed the most is Israel, where it is very well established in the National Health Insurance. Dr Howard Tandeter describes the development of family medicine in Israel, with a focus on the programmes taught in the Department of Family Medicine of Ben-Gurion University of the Negev, concluding that Israeli family medicine is one of the most experienced and pioneering in the world. (Tandeter, 2007)

This National Health Insurance was enshrined in law on 1 January 1995, it is universal (with a guarantee of quality medical attention for all residents), obligatory and egalitarian. These outlined principles are guaranteed by the following factors: the service provider may not know the price paid by the user (guarantee of equality); the rivalry that occurs as much between providers as well as family doctors due to the free choice of family doctor and provider (HMO); by the fact that each patient has total access to any medical information about them (guarantee of quality provision of services); that the system is based in family medicine, and that doctors of this specialism work full-time, are paid *per capita*, are completely dedicated to patients, and able to fit in a university teaching career through research (guarantee of quality medical attention); that fiscal decentralisation exists at all levels, which ensures that lenders seek resource optimisation (performance efficiency guarantee), and that quality control at all levels is institutionalised. (Kahan, 2007)

Many people ask about the difference between a family doctor and a GP (or General Practitioner). A health issues article entitled "Family Physician vs. General Practitioner" expresses that difference with great clarity: "On the surface, an FP can seem very similar to a general practitioner […] both can be considered primary care physicians. However, a family physician has received more specialized training in family medicine than a general practitioner. […] Family physicians are required to receive 3 years practical experience (or residency) [while] general practitioners, on the other hand, may only be required to have completed one year of residency before they can be certified." (Pregnancy-Info.Net. 2016.) In Israel the required period of residency to obtain the title of family doctor is 4 years, with internships in primary care clinics, hospitals and public care sites.

During a two-year rotation in community clinics, the resident's experience and teaching focuses on the treatment of the individual, family dynamics, psychosocial factors, preventative medicine and medical practice organisation. The principal objectives of medical residency are: focus of medical attention and care according to the natural history of the disease (of every disease), obtaining updated knowledge in clinical practice, paediatrics, gynaecology, surgery, psychiatry and public health, analysing cost effectiveness in order to inform decision making, employing the principle of advice, and management of the legal-social, economic and work-related aspects of illnesses. Needless to say, this family doctor must possess efficient and clinical communication tools in order to establish treatment and follow-up programmes in primary, secondary and tertiary care that are specific to each patient and in line with the necessities of the corresponding family and social context. (See Analysis of Paradox 68)

To conclude my brief analysis of the 89th Paradox: *Family medicine vs. Community medicine*, I choose the illustrative and exemplary list of values published in the Policy and Procedure Manual of the Hennepin County Medical Center Family Medicine Residency Program 2012–2013:

- Excellence in Medical Care: Care that is based on the best medical knowledge and evidence.
- Dignity and Compassion.
- Whole Person: Promoting health and healing that addresses body, mind, spirit, family and community.
- Cultural Respect: Providing care that is responsive to people's unique cultural characteristics such as race, ethnicity, national origin, language, gender, age, religion, sexual orientation, and physical disability.
- Health of All: Valuing healthy people, families, and communities. Working to optimize the health of all people and to eliminate health disparities.
- Physician Wellness: Embracing healthy living for residents.

REFERENCES
1   *Organización Mundial de Médicos de Familia.* 1996. Mexico. Bol. Med. Fam. 4 (1): 9
2   *La contribución del médico de familia.* 1996. Mexico. Bol. Med. Fam. 4 (1): 1–8
3   Longlett S. K., Kruse J. E., Wesley R. M. 2001. *Community-Oriented Primary Care: Historical Perspective.* American Board of Family Practice. 14 (1): 54–63
4   Kahan E. Editorial. 2007. *Artículo dedicado a la Medicina Familia en Israel.* Mexico. Arch en Med Fam 9 (1): 11–16
5   Tandeter H. 2007. *Family Medicine in Israel: A National Overview and Examples from Ben-Gurion University in the Negev.* Mexico. Arch en Med Fam 9 (1): 65–70

6   PregnancyInfo.Net. 2016. *Family Practitioners* (Online) (Accessed 9 May 2016) Available from:
    <http://www.pregnancyinfo.net/family_practitioners.html>

7   Hennepin County Medical Center Family Medicine Residency Program. 2013. *Policy and Procedure Manual of the Hennepin County Medical Center Family Medicine Residency Program 2012–2013* (Online) (Accessed 10 May 2016) Available from:
    <http://residents.fammed.org/Manuals/Policy%20Manual%202012-13up-dated%208-13.pdf>

JOSÉ FÉLIX OLETTA

I am honoured that you have permitted me to read the new extended edition of your book *Medical Paradoxes*.

Allow me to congratulate you first and foremost for an accomplished piece of work that summarises your reflections on a number of fundamental issues for medicine of our time, and of the challenges for the medicine of the future, both as a profession and for the good of society.

You have aptly chosen the paradox as your literary means. You use the multiple meanings of words to highlight contrasts, thereby drawing attention to diverse and only recently considered questions; you disentangle these questions in your narrative by clarifying their meaning or by analysing key information or ideas.

The word paradox derives from the Latin form *paradoxum*, which is a loan from the Greek *paradoxon* "unexpected, incredible, unique", etymologically formed of the preposition para-, which means "next to" or "beside" plus the root *doxon* "opinion, good judgement".

Your use of the paradox is undoubtedly a powerful stimulus for reflection. Philosophers often use paradoxes to reveal the complexity of reality. The paradox also permits a demonstration of the limits of the tools of the human mind. The identification of paradoxes within concepts that at first glance appear to be simple and reasonable has

293

driven important advances in science, philosophy and mathematics. Medicine as an inexact science does not escape this effect.

Throughout your essay one finds diverse opportunities to develop the debate on many different medical paradoxes. Perhaps the most prominent by their nature are those that circle around topics of ethical medicine, where contrasts, contradictions and unresolved dilemmas arise. Some are true paradoxes, others antinomies by definition, others conditional, in fact, others probabilistic or statistical.

What is certain is that you invite us throughout your writing to make correct use of the mind's capacity for abstraction in order to achieve an adequate comprehension of the aforementioned paradoxes. A good understanding of paradoxes and their explanations contributes to one's personal development of the capacity for analysis, for processing abstract information and occasionally a growth in intellect, without any philosophical intention.

You mention some aporias, which refer to reasoning in which contradictions or unresolved paradoxes arise, questions without answers; in such cases the aporias emerge as logical difficulties, almost always of a speculative nature, but also in the Socratic sense by which we liberate ourselves from false knowledge. It leaves the way open and gives us the confidence to understand that these unresolved paradoxes have been resolved thanks to cognitive advances or changes of paradigm, of world view, or episteme.

The style you employ throughout your 100 Medical Paradoxes and your "Quo vadis medicine?" chapter recalls that of G. K. Chesterton (1874–1936), known as "The Prince of Paradoxes"; one senses the influence of this writer, who expressed his opinions with a polemic air and not a little humour, when you sensitively describe these paradoxes as part of the adventures of a long and fruitful life.

Chesterton would begin his writings with a statement that appeared to be most normal, but would then make us realise that things are not as they seem, and that many things are said without being thought through in any depth. It is worth noting that he always maintained that argument in its Latin denomination is *reductio ad absurdum*.

He fought tooth and nail everything that he considered a modern error: rationalism and scientism, he opposed common sense and faith, the cruelty of the industrial civilisation and capitalist interests, the social ideal.

In his search for the truth, Chesterton came up against many obstacles, but he always maintained an open mind and would not be detained by these walls unless he was convinced that they had to be torn down in order to continue with his search: "Whenever you remove any fence, always pause long enough to ask yourself, 'Why was it put there in the first place?'"

Paraphrasing Chesterton's criticism of the Catholic Church's conservatism: "they didn't want a Church that adapted to the times, as human beings remain the same and need guidance: We do not really want a religion that is right where we are right. What we want is a religion that is right where we are wrong . . ." (Chesterton, 1926)

It could be said that your criticisms of conservatism in medicine in some paradoxes equates to stating: "We don't really want a Medicine that is right where we are right. What we want is a Medicine that is right where we are wrong."

Just like medicine, over the course of its two thousand years the Catholic religion as a secular institution has covered all experiences and nearly all mistakes. According to Chesterton the result was:

". . . a map in which all the blind alleys and bad roads are clearly marked, all the ways that have been shown to be worthless by the best of all evidence: the evidence of those who have gone down them". (Chesterton, 1926)

Perhaps this is one of the keys to the doors that open on to the path to truth, light and certainty; which could mark out the medical "ethos" of the initiated of this profession, erase the darkness of uncertainty and the current crisis in the profession, which is driven by internal and external causes, in a world in transition towards a revolution of knowledge, communication and globalisation, in which you state:

"*[Medical tradition is] an almost impossible obstacle to overcome for those forces attempting to convert medical practice into a mere exercise of sophisticated technology. This separates the interests of the generation that provided the knowledge to inspire said technology, from the inventiveness of the same and from its administration in the society that it serves.*"

We agree with your statement:

"*[We must] consider how to resolve potential conflicts and gain a shrewd understanding of the challenges generated by these paradoxes:*

- *The challenge of accepting, studying and correcting the criticism that has been made of medicine, when any support or justification is found, even when the justification often appears to be exaggerated or manipulated.*
- *The challenge of resolving evident contradictions in the art of practising medicine.*
- *The challenge of appreciating and taking advantage of the great benefits of scientific research, applying them wisely to the management of illness, without losing sight of their implicit limitations and the permanent balancing act that must occur between the technological and humanist component in medicine, where facultative behaviour must always be regulated, so that the act of medicine does not lose its true meaning.*

My greatest appreciation and admiration for your work.

REFERENCES
1   Chesterton, G. K. 1926. *The Catholic Church and Conversion* (Online) (Accessed 10 May 2016) Available from: <http://www.cse.dmu.ac.uk/~mward/gkc/books/conversion.txt>
2   Chesterton, G. K. 2014. *Why I am a Catholic.* (Online) (Accessed 10 May 2016) Available from: <http://www.chesterton.org/why-i-am-a-catholic/>

EDUARDO MATHISON

Your presentation is spectacular. I am convinced that health is as much an economical activity as any other, although much more complex; medical knowledge is indispensible to its production and operation, but without financial and managerial control and knowledge it is hard pushed to be successful.

JOSÉ FÉLIX PATIÑO

The title of your excellent work concerns me a little: *Paradoxes.* Are they not rather Contradictions, Dilemmas, Crossroads?

Paradox
The RAE Dictionary (*Real Academia Española* – Royal Spanish Academy) says the following: paradox (from the Latin paradoxus, and this from the Gr. παράδοξα 1. Adj. Obs. **Paradoxical 2.** n. Idea that is strange or opposite to common opinion and feeling. **3.** n. Implausible or absurd assertion, which is presented under the guise of truth **4.** n. Rhet. Figure of thought that consists in employing expressions or phrases that contain contradiction. *Look at the miser, poor in his wealth.*

Dilemma
(From the Lat. *dilemma*, and this from the Greek δίλημμα, de δι, dos, & 'premisa'.) **1.** n. Argument formed of two disjunctively opposite

propositions in such arrangement that if either of the two is denied or accepted, what is intended to be proved is demonstrated. 2. n. Doubt, quandary.

Contradiction

(From the Lat. contradictio, -ōnis.) 1. n. Action or effect of contradicting. 2. n. Affirmation and denial that oppose and destroy each other reciprocally. 3. n. opposition (contrariety). Involve, or implicate, – a proposition or assertion. 1. Locs. Verb. Containing contradictory things. Entry 4 of the RAE's definition of *Paradox* justifies the use of the term *paradoxes*, but think about it a little more.

My observations:

9th Paradox: Family doctors vs. Specialists

Yes, the general practitioner is the backbone of any health system. They are also the gatekeeper (which is a role that can become disoriented in systems of managed care, like in Colombia where the doctor becomes a goalkeeper). But in our countries, general practitioner training leaves much to be desired. Here in Colombia one is a general practitioner when one graduates, and there are no post-graduates! In the United Kingdom that you know so well, general practitioner training is between 5–7 years.

10th Paradox: The right to health vs. The right to medical attention

I do believe it is correct to say the right to health, given that the term health goes way beyond medical attention: preventative medicine, collective and individual public health, healthy lifestyle … In the face of the ominous advance of managed care (disastrous in Colombia), health as a fundamental right consecrated in national political constitutions is an important achievement. Frankly, I believe that this deserves your profound re-consideration. See 22nd Paradox further on.

20th Paradox: Insurance institutions vs. The medical profession

I consider that greater depth would be fitting here, as managed care has not only failed in the United States, but also thunderously so in Colombia. The introduction of the business-minded intermediary is a contradiction of social morality. Healthcare should be social, with insurers offering additional policies to those who can afford them. Financial intermediation destroyed the healthcare system in Colombia and we now find ourselves in an extremely difficult situation.

22nd Paradox: Politicians vs. The medical profession

In Colombia, health has been established constitutionally as a fundamental human right. This has translated into governmental efforts to guarantee that right, with two pieces of legislation currently being discussed: the Statutory Law already passed by Congress and now being studied by the Constitutional Court, and an act of ordinary Law that was passed in Senate but got stuck in Chamber due to fierce opposition from all healthcare sectors, from patient organisations to wide sectors of society. What they are pursuing is a healthcare system that guarantees this right through due attention, prevention and rehabilitation. As your book will be read in all countries, I suggest you edit this Paradox in a different way, recognising that in other countries healthcare is considered a fundamental right.

23rd Paradox: Rational use vs. Abusive and convenient use of intensive care units

Very good, allow me to suggest the importance of legislating a signed and witnessed Advance Directive to be duly distributed by hospitals. This has resolved the problem here on numerous occasions. At the Santa Fe Foundation in Bogotá we also have a Hospital Ethics Committee that checks absurd cases taken to ICUs. It is common for families covered by the General Health System Social Security to take along people of advanced age, including those with Alzheimer's and other clinical conditions that render them absent, because it is more convenient to put them into an ICU than look after them at home. In our experience, the convenience factor favours the families, not the doctors.

34th Paradox: The truth vs. The partial truth

Here perhaps you should include information given to oncology patients, including any results to be expected from therapy, and their prognosis. I have found it very beneficial to be able to say to some cancer patients that their disease is no longer a mortal disease, but a chronic one.

35th Paradox: Hippocratic medicine vs. Iatrogenesis

The Institute of Medicine publication *To Err is Human* and the numbers it includes have caused real damage to the medical profession. It doesn't acknowledge William Osler's statement from a hundred years ago that medicine is the art of managing uncertainty, nor does it acknowledge chaos theory, which refers to complex non-linear and adaptive systems, like human beings, who manifest unpredictable behaviour due to the laws of physics or statistics. I emphatically believe that these should not be called medical errors, but rather unexpected occurrences or events.

ARTURO RAMOS CALDERA

Reading the book was thrilling, entertaining and interesting, which is why I believe its publication will fill an important gap in the overall training of all students of medicine. Even when an in-depth analysis of each and every one of its topics is not attempted (which would be impossible to achieve), the simple act of listing them and of citing a bibliography for each one offers an overall view for the reader and a first guide to dig deeper into those that most interest them.

PABLO A PULIDO

Well done on your work on *Medical Paradoxes*! Allow me to congratulate you once again.

Medical practice has certainly changed, and the surroundings that influence it even more so. Professionals have to learn to work in a complex system.

The challenge is clearly enormous; it requires teamwork, which is one of the reasons why our founding institutions are extremely relevant.

This is clearly a new and complex situation with new dynamics amidst a changing reality, into which the medical profession should intelligently and creatively intervene, above all those Medical Academies and Public Health Institutions responsible for professional training and the preservation of the ethical values that make a well-perceived medical professionalism possible. The medical profession should respond to its fundamental objective, which is none other than the patient's health and that of the community it serves.

RAÚL SANZ MACHADO

Hello, my friend, these Medical Paradoxes of yours are admirable, as much for their content as for the meticulous research with which you support them. Although ignorant of this material, I am honoured that you have sought my opinions and recommendations, which I offer with the necessary care and diligence. Save yourself the modesty of calling it a "little book", it is an excellent work that provokes deep reflection. Congratulations.

The introduction includes a number of paradoxes, as a preamble to general concepts, such as:

Cost of Medical Services

1. In order to form an opinion on value, the fundamental principle of the science of "marketing" should be applied. According to this principle, the greater the demand for goods or consumer services, the greater the investment-production, and the greater production and competitiveness. The trend dictates the adjustment of final costs to reasonable levels that are sufficient to guarantee quality of services, barring those economic factors of inflation or insufficient foreign currency that have a negative impact on desirable supply levels, as has systematically occurred in recent years in Venezuela. When supply exceeds demand, in quality and quantity, prices tend to be low. As the popular Venezuelan saying goes: *No hay pele* – you can't go wrong.

2. Medawar's argument according to which "laboratory tests remain the scientific property of medicine", certainly is paradoxical. In effect, these days thorough diagnosis of physical ailments is impossible without the help of patient organ investigations via the advanced technological and scientific systems and means available, such as those in the field known as "biological engineering".

3. Worldwide population. Population growth has already reached 7,000 million inhabitants, the equivalent of seven times more than the population of the first 1,000 million registered in the relatively brief period of 184 years from 1830–2013. Notwithstanding the population increase, in the XIX and XX centuries there has also been a significant increase in victims of disasters, epidemics, tragedies, military conflicts, hunger, abortion and crime, although not in the same proportion, as well as increasing threats to the environment and biosphere. These serious threats to humanity are certainly just cause for concern on the part of experts, demographic scientists, with it being paradoxical that "man

who creates human life and defends it with his scientific advances is also he who destroys it" (drugs, tobacco, alcoholism, famine, environmental damage, etc.).

1st Paradox: The science of medicine vs. The art of medicine

The discovery of new drugs, treatments and medical concepts continue to evolve, bringing innovative scientific and surgical advances capable of improving and prolonging quality of life. There are projects in experimental phase that foretell possibilities that were inconceivable until now, especially in the field of "medical engineering" and the curing of illnesses considered to be irreversible. In spite of everything, environmental contamination and damage, dietary habits, sedentary lifestyles and daily stress contribute to the deterioration of life and a generation of fatal diseases.

2nd Paradox: Demographic explosion vs. Quality of life

The empirical medical treatment given to Simón Bolívar in San Pedro Alejandrino in the final stages of his life, as described in the medical sections of the diary of his "doctor" Dr Alejandro P. Reverend, demonstrates that the application of poultices, potions, purgatives, enemas, etc. were not only incapable of improving the patient's health, but in fact contributed to worsening his debilitation and shortened the final stages of his life. However, over the course of the centuries, the doctors of old, such as Galen who along with Hippocrates was considered the maximum authority on medical practice in his time and the father of medicine, the legendary doctor Asclepius, God of Greek mythology, or the alchemists determined to find the "panacea" capable of curing any illness, have contributed principles that are considered fundamental to medical science.

To the pharmacological properties of any medication, one would have to add regularisation of the application of its properties, taking into account that its frequent or permanent consumption or application could be counterproductive to health.

The Fleming Case

Sir William Osler's statement in which he diminishes the discoverer of penicillin does not seem fair. The application of a medication or medical procedure is as valuable as the person who invented or discovered it. In the mid-twentieth century, through an "unexpected and fortunate error", Alexander Fleming discovered the fungus *Penicillium notatum*, which when scientifically modified became penicillin, the first broad-spectrum antibiotic, which has saved the lives of thousands of millions of human beings. The benefits to life resulting from scientific development enjoyed by human beings today would have been impossible without the pioneering contributions of long ago.

The Right To Health

The right to health, consecrated in the National Constitution, is both a product and consequence of quality, timely and appropriate pharmaceutical supplies and materials, and medical and hospital resources. These are indispensible for health, especially within the marginal socio-economical class, which is one of the largest and severest shortcomings of government policies.

Curare in Anaesthesia

The muscular relaxant properties of curare were discovered in the middle of the past century in Venezuelan Guyana by scientists from Abbott Laboratories in the USA, when they realised that local indigenous tribes paralysed the respiratory system of animals by using arrows covered in curare, a plant substance that did not have the same effect on those who ate the animal's meat. Abbott initiated experiments in the '30s and '40s and managed to isolate the active property *Tubocurarine*, thereby producing the injectable muscle relaxant product, which is used successfully in the reduction of bone fractures.

Transplants

I would have to add: locomotive limbs, prosthesis, as well as other variants: DNA, ultrasonography, bone MRI to investigate metastatic cancer, etc.

3rd Paradox: Vegetative life vs. Euthanasia

As you state, given that the brain is the master of all organs, it should be understood that this is not a "brain transplant", but rather the "transplant of a human body to a brain", one of the greatest future trials in medical science due to the challenges and consequences that it implicates. I would have to add that advancements in technology and electronics have made possible the brains and robots classified as "intelligent".

The "right to die" (Euthanasia) and the "right to life" (of the unborn) continue to be complex disputes in ethical, moral, legal and religious terms, because the decision in both cases does not ultimately depend on the conscious free will of the victim, rather on the "victimiser" who is the "judge" of both rights. There is undisputable evidence of cases of rehabilitation in people previously declared terminally ill, cases that are inexplicable to science, which only confirm the complexity of the matter. And so . . . ?

4th Paradox: Economic weakness or need vs. Quality of medical attention

It is also worth highlighting cases such as the High Cost Medication Pharmacy, Social Security's commendable initiative, a first-rate service that provides high cost, non-tradable pharmaceuticals, imported by Obligatory Social Security, and donated to patients affected by cancer,

AIDs, and other diseases, even if they don't have SSO pension or benefits (subject to medical report and prescription). The stock availability and comfort this efficient service offers to patients are particularly noteworthy.

5th Paradox: Lies vs. State secrets

There ought to be public awareness about the health of leaders and senior public officials, as is the case in the majority of democracies. Here one could apply the popular wise saying: "If you have nothing to hide, you have nothing to fear." Within the history of Venezuelan presidents, the case of President Hugo Chavez and the media manipulation or concealment of the truth about his health, contrasts with that of other Heads of State like Cipriano Castro, Juan Vicente Gómez and Diógenes Escalante, amongst others, whose states of health were made known to the public through timely medical reports.

6th Paradox: Consuming alcohol vs. Good health

It would appear that there is a decrease in alcohol addiction, compared with an incremental increase in drug addiction, which according to WHO figures affects more than 300 million people, of whom the majority are young people, adolescents even. The Uruguayan government's initiative to legalise marijuana use, even in a restrictive way, raises serious issues, much in the same way as with abortion. We know how it begins, but not how it will end.

7th Paradox: Organ donation vs. Sale of organs for transplant

The sale of human organs (which is different to voluntary donation) is a moral issue, when one compares the donor, who profits financially from the situation, with the patient, whose "right to life" benefits.

8th Paradox: Staying in one's country of origin vs. Emigration

The growing migration of human resources and Venezuelan families is most definitely a consequence of internal factors attributable to the failure of government policies, insecurity and unemployment in the first decade of this century. This is in evident contrast with the immigration wave of skilled workers, from Spain and Colombia especially, in the times of the Pérez Jiménez government.

9th Paradox: Family doctors vs. Specialists

The "family doctor" was common in the first decades of the past century, when house calls from doctors were customary. Where appropriate, patients would be referred to a specialist. Laboratory research and radiology prior to a diagnosis were not common until the progressive evolution of scientific resources. (During my childhood, I recall house calls, doctor's bags in hand, from family doctors of the standing of Gustavo H. Machado and Hernández Zozaya)

10th Paradox: The right to health vs. The right to medical attention

Given the clear incapacity of the State to appropriately and efficiently accomplish such principles, the *right to health*, consecrated in the National Constitution, just like the guarantee of personal security and life, will be nothing more than a "dead letter". The head of State's repeated declaration "I assume my responsibility" is meaningless, a mere demagogic statement. Besides the doubtful nature and questionable suitability of the medical resources brought over from Cuba, with no respect for the qualifications referred to in the Constitution or Schools of Medicine regulations, the fact remains that guaranteeing the correct provision and administration of services, hospitals and health centres requires doctors and personnel specialised in hospital management and the adequate provision of supplies and resources by the State.

307

Proof of this is the case of the failure of one of the most important medical hospital centres in Caracas, which was paralysed for a number of years due to serious financial and administrative problems caused by a lack of managerial experience. Thanks to a total reorganisation of the project, now in capable hands, this medical hospital centre is today a model of its kind in Latin America.

11th Paradox: Fair fees vs. Abusive fees

Fees for medical services and support in Venezuela are by comparison significantly lower than in the USA, Europe and other countries. Furthermore, many doctors of recognised prestige offer their services for free to non-profit institutions on a weekly basis. A notable example is the Federico Ozanam Medical Healthcare Centre, sponsored, administered and operated by the Foundation of the same name since 1996, at the initiative of the San Vicente de Paul Foundation, which was created by businessman Jacob Dib (deceased), and currently under the direction of his direct descendants. Based in Guarenas, it is an excellent non-profit institution, with no economic support from the government, equipped with all services, specialisations, hospital facilities, emergency facilities and scientific and technological medical resources. Run by around a hundred doctors with more than 40 specialisms in medicine and deontology, it operates under a *social solidarity* model, through which those patients not covered by Security or any form of pre-paid medicine, pay for their care according to their means, with many being partially or total exempt from payment. In 2013, more than 150,000 patients received assistance in the order of a total of 2,380,000 bolivars. In other countries, the pre-paid medicine system is a "good business" because its rates are linked to the good health of its members, permitting a reduction in operative costs.

12th Paradox: Doctors vs. Lawyers

Generally, rates of legal services will have greater breadth due to their professional and commercial character, often taking into account the client's economic means, the complexity of the case and man hours required by the matters that fall within their expertise. However, the standing and reputation of the law firm will also affect the rates.

13th Paradox: Reproductive medicine vs. Reproductive manipulation

Obviously these cases are of a specific and complex nature and will, in cases of abortion or euthanasia, depend on the patient or relatives. Given that they concern Moral and Ethical Law they cannot always be resolved through legal channels.

14th Paradox: Employees vs. Administrators

In addition to my comments on Paradox 10, in order to guarantee the quality of doctor-hospital services, integration between medical and administrative roles should be inseparable. In Venezuela, the general absence of dedicated management is the predominant cause of the dismal performance of public health. This is aggravated by repeated shortages in medical resources and instruments, which cause a constant undesirable "back-and-forthing" of patients, frequently resulting in deaths in emergency situations and absences of appropriate aid. It is inexplicable that institutions like the Institute of Social Security, or the Ministry of Health, are directed and operated by "politicians" or friends of people in office. The results are more than telling. There are a number of exceptions in the Institute of Social Security, the successful post of Dr José Luis Silva Luongo (deceased), an expert in insurance and the ex-Minister of Finance, as well as Dr Rafael Rísquez Iribarren (deceased), not forgetting the prominent figures of Doctors Arnoldo Gabaldón, Martín Vegas, Espíritu Santo Mendoza and Enrique Tejera, amongst others.

15th Paradox: The medical act: Complete vs. Partial

Needless to say, a medical specialist, aware of their personal competence and out of respect for their professional standing cannot nor should not just accept the opposing opinions of their superiors regarding diagnosis and medical practice. In such cases, an ad hoc board, at the Medical College or ultimately at the judicial authority, would evaluate these cases, but even then, I believe that it is the treating doctor's "judgement call".

16th Paradox: Clinic vs. Laboratory

Here the idea of deliberation based on knowledge and experience seem reasonable, as reflected in the wise colloquial saying: "Ni tanto que queme al santo, ni tan poco que no lo alumbre" which could be translated as "Don't light up the saint so much that they burn, but not so little that they are not illuminated".* In other words "don't over-egg the pudding", find a balance.

17th Paradox: Essential examinations vs. Optional examinations

My observation in the previous paradox is certainly applicable here too. There are cases in which the treating doctor takes examinations and tests to the extreme, beyond what is reasonably necessary, as if to "cure with health" and protect against potential diagnostic or medical practice errors.

18th Paradox: Satisfaction vs. Dissatisfaction in medical practice

The frequent cases of dissatisfaction with services and cases of professional incompetence could be the result of an abhorrent legal and constitutional violation. A reliance on the services of the tens of thousands of "doctors", with no or insufficient academic merits unfulfilling of

* Translator's note: This refers to the candles that are lit before images of Saints in Catholic churches.

obligatory national qualifications or the Medical College Code of Conduct, imported by the national government has led to frequent and grave consequences over the last decade. This has perverted the objective of the Barrio Adentro Mission, whose implementation in surgeries and clinics in poor areas, many of which are inoperative, has been generally deplorable. The growing number of Cuban "doctors" who have chosen to emigrate to other countries is significant.

19th Paradox: Traditional information vs. Information sourced from the Internet

The remarkable level of information about diseases and treatments available via the internet, television networks and other means, sometimes from unqualified sources set out to make a profit, promotes and incites the undesirable practice of self-medication, which could be counter-productive and even aggravate symptoms. Suffice to cite the recent cases of breast implants that have resulted in legal claims, and the application of rejuvenating substances (botox and others), which have subsequently been prohibited due to the damage caused. These kinds of "virtual medical consultations" should be strictly regulated, like in previous decades, when doctors and health professionals abstained from using the media to inform, declare or make generalised diagnoses, let alone prescribe pharmaceuticals, including vitamins and over-the-counter medications.

Note the continued lack of information in newspapers and other media about the contents, properties, dosages and applications of exclusive medical prescriptions; this is as a result of laboratories and manufacturing companies protecting product confidentiality. As we know, this information, especially with regards to new products, is periodically transmitted to doctors in person by "visiting doctors", who also offer advice and product samples. Those listed as products of "free sale" without prescription, are widely advertised, and in the majority of cases are not prescribed by doctors, for obvious reasons. The frequent TV interviews with specialist doctors, which most certainly influence patients, are clearly just about publicity.

20th Paradox: Insurance institutions vs. The medical profession

Although medical insurance against malpractice claims protects the doctor in the USA against potential lawsuits, as you have noted, it has an exorbitant effect on the level of fees, with a double impact for the patient who partially assumes the insurance cost in the fees they pay, but may also suffer from the consequences of any potentially irreparable damage caused. In European countries with "socialised medicine", the health service is often impeccable and what's more cost free, even for tourists and non-residents, although its equivalent is necessarily reflected in the compulsory tax regime paid by all citizens.

21st Paradox: The pharmaceutical industry vs. The medical profession

Pharmaceutical companies operate like any other private profit-seeking industry, but with a focus on charitable or hospital organisations. A recent CNN report looked at the issue of new advanced technology medications currently being researched or even ready for sale. Faced with the possibility or conviction that these medications could contribute to the cure of traditional or incurable illnesses, the companies tend to delay their launch while generally numerous stocks of alternative medications run out, which could be considered unethical. This also happens with the prescription of "brand" medication, which is significantly more expensive than "generic" brands, although stocks of these in the market-place seem to be higher, due to the number of patients looking for a saving.

22nd Paradox: Politicians vs. The medical profession

The clear managerial inability of the State to adequately supply hospitals and public health centres means that it is not possible for them to guarantee the constitutional right of health. From this ineffectiveness, it can be deduced that for the government public health is a "burden", that it is not a particular priority, except when it comes to making electoral promises.

23rd Paradox: Rational use vs. Abusive and convenient use of intensive care units

Clearly, recourse to intensive care has its pros and cons; the advantages, interests and benefits are in the doctors' favour to the detriment of the patients, although this does not mean a lack in the quality of services. This characteristic is also observed in medical consultation services. As there is no scheduled consultation appointment system, due in part to patients not turning up for appointments, consultations are allocated on a first-come-first-served basis, which generates long waiting times, at times up to an hour or more, but this system suits the doctors. On top of this there is the outrage of costly non-essential additional examinations and the difficulty, even impossibility, of post-consultation communication with the doctor, some of whom will delegate this role to their secretary or nurse who liaises on their behalf. However, we must recognise cases of exception such as the excellent service offered by the Arsuve Oncology Group at the La Floresta Medical Centre, which has its headquarters at the La Trinidad Teaching Medical Centre. In addition to their comfortable and modern facilities, they also offer direct communication with their doctors. Finally, we should also mention the insensitive obligation to pay for services in advance.

26th Paradox: Humility vs. Arrogance and dogma

The case of Dr Favaloro is extremely powerful and dramatic. It confirms the biblical saying "No man is a prophet in his own land". One can only imagine what his career path might have been in the international arena had he stayed in the USA or the European Union, like the cases of outstanding Venezuelan scientists and doctors, from Baruch Benacerraf (Nobel Prize for Medicine) and the "Wizard of Pipe" Humberto Fernández Morán, to our era when the *marabino** engineer Rafael Reid, a graduate of the University of Carabobo, achieved the presidency of the prestigious MIT in Boston through his enlightened merits.

27th Paradox: The right to life vs. The right to abortion

We need hardly reaffirm that human and animal life scientifically begin with the fertilisation of an egg in the maternal uterus, that is how, according to evolutionary theory, organic life originated from the emergence of some amino-acid or protein, a stellar primary micro-organism, millions of years ago. An organism-being originates from the fertilisation of the maternal ovary, transforming into a foetus endowed with its own genetic code or map (DNA), as well as vital organs, body, mind, heart, etc. and a soul, a spiritual identity. Therefore, in my personal opinion, the life of an unborn is and must be unconditionally impenetrable. It is as human in the maternal womb as it is after birth. Without understanding the complexity of the issue, nobody has the right to be a "judge", making life or death decisions. Experience has shown the existence of cases of human beings declared to be "brain dead" recovering their lives after many years of vegetative existence. The supernatural transcends being human.

28th Paradox: Social security vs. Private medicine

Only in countries with an advanced culture of social security (USA, European Union, Asia) does social security in the hands of the State

* Translator's note: *marabino* indicates somebody from the north-east of Venezuela.

314

really work, in comparison with the deplorable and often corrupt situation in other countries, especially in Latin America and Africa where social security either doesn't exist or suffers from serious defects and scientific, operative and ethical shortcomings. In Venezuela, *Seguro Social Obligatorio* (SSO – Obligatory Social Security) and the Ministry of Health, upon which public aid and social security services depend, are shameful examples of ineptitude, corruption and an absence of any management or administrative structure. By way of example, one only needs to cite the unquantifiable debt of public bodies that deduct monthly SSO premiums from workers, but do not then pass them onto the *Instituto Venezolano de los Seguros Sociales* (IVSS – Institute of Social Security).

30th Paradox: Clinical medicine vs. Molecular medicine
In spite of Dr James Le Fanu's dissenting opinion, DNA has been one of the most fundamental instruments for human identification, especially in the criminology sphere. In my view, the issue would be in the possible and unknown mysteries that DNA still holds.

31st Paradox: The triumphs vs. The failures of contemporary medicine
As far as cancer treatments are concerned, scientific research still has much to achieve, above all in the relief of patients' reactions to chemotherapy, like general malaise and alopecia.

32nd Paradox: Pain and power vs. Medicine and money
Paradoxically, it seems unquestionable that half (at the very least) of what a patient spends on health will only serve to prolong human life, which poses the axiom "the longer the life expectancy, the greater the economical benefit". At the end of the day, the price of obtaining consolation for a patient's family is often very high.

33rd Paradox. Local medicine vs. Global medicine

Undoubtedly, the health of the third world population is predominately in the hands of countries that are more advanced in research and medical science; however, the overall solution to improving quality of life in Latin America and other world regions lies with medical training and the incorporation of those educational, scientific and technical resources required to guarantee corrective action. Preventative education through the spread of better behaviour, attitudes, habits, hygiene, diet, environmental conditions (drinkable water, rubbish and waste water disposal), all of which are clearly lacking in countries where marginality is prevalent, are also indispensible.

Paradox 35. Hippocratic medicine vs. Iatrogenesis

Besides human frailty in medical practice and Iatrogenesis, it is evident which critical values should prevail in a strict and complete scientific and professional training of medical human resources (including paramedical and auxiliary resources). This eradicates the mediocrity and absence of skills and competency that result from the irresponsible training that a number of graduates favour over scientific training, catering to disgraceful political and demagogic interests. To have conceived of and accepted a system of mass education of thousands of "doctors", comprised of barely 3 years training and doubtful or no academic practice whatsoever, is unacceptable. Moreover, if any profession demands qualified teachers with post-graduate training and proven medical or surgical experience, it is medicine, because nothing less than human life is at stake. Suffice to mention the failure of Barrio Adentro (in spite of the good intentions that drove its creation), where tens of thousands of doctors were imported from Cuba, without indispensible qualifications, training or medical practice experience.

37th Paradox: Curative medicine vs. Hygiene

Curative medicine along with hygiene habits and environmental sanitation are as significantly important as the prevention of contagious diseases; this material should be heavily included in school curricula at all levels. Ignorance in matters of preventative healthcare is prevalent in marginal socio-economic classes and areas, where there is a clear deterioration in public health. Governmental policies are, or should be, significantly pertinent.

39th Paradox: Fashions in medicine vs. Immutable truths

The abundance of novelty, preventative and curative treatments, supposed doctors' testimonies and promoted "promises" ("Satisfaction guaranteed or your money back") within the advertorial avalanche deployed by manufacturers is mainly the result of profit-seeking behaviour and an attempted seduction of consumers. Until recently, natural medications like Ginkgo Biloba, Glucosamine, multi-vitamins "for fatigue, stress and weakened mental faculties", slimming drugs, amongst many others were in "fashion". Proper regulation and moderation of the indiscriminate circulation of the properties and use of such medications would be preferable.

40th Paradox: The battle against illness vs. The battle against death

The strategic key to a healthy increased life expectancy is "maintenance", much like the maintenance of industrial plants, equipment, machinery and vehicles. Not in vain has it been stated that the human organism is the most perfect "machine" ever invented. None other is capable of functioning uninterruptedly for 70 to 80 consecutive years or more. Physical and mental exercise, good everyday habits, appropriate diet and a calm attitude when faced with the inevitable tensions of current life, as well as the invigorating effect of cohabitation and peace, are all factors that benefit health and "advanced" youth. The celebrated French 18th-century thinker Denis Diderot said: "Doctors are always working to preserve our health and cooks to destroy it, but the latter are the more often successful." I fear that he may be right.

64th Paradox: Freud's psychoanalysis vs. Neuropharmacy

The stress, daily aggression, and violence that generate emotional instability and depression in human behaviour have made anti-depressants, psychotropic medication and similar products one of the largest pharmacology markets in the world, in spite of the fact that the purchase of many of them requires a doctor's prescription.

65th Paradox: The criminalisation of certain drugs vs. General use of the same or similar drugs

The recent legalisation of the sale and consumption of marijuana in Uruguay, notwithstanding the imposed restrictions, has consequently awoken worldwide expectations including within organisations such as the WHO, FDA, DEA, CIA etc., which suggests that this practice will be generalised, in spite of the fact that in Holland and other countries it is already a fact. In Scandinavian countries too there are designated areas (public squares and parks) for drug enthusiasts. However, it's also foreseeable that growing consumption and irregular sale of marijuana may stimulate the risk of "hard" drug use, a consequence of addiction, especially in adolescents.

66th Paradox: Prolongation of life vs. Quality of life

To your excellent and correct analysis, I would only add that the emotional flipside of aspiring to a long and healthy life is the other needs that it causes, the increased number of services and inevitable increase in costs produced by a prolonged geriatric period. With bitter humour we recall the witty advice given on the occasion of somebody's birthday: "If you keep getting older, you'll die . . ." In any case, it would be better to keep celebrating the anniversary of your birth.

318

67th Paradox: Lifestyle diseases vs. Environmental diseases

One might ask if diseases, as a consequence of bodily decline and natural death, the worrying exponential growth of deaths from violence, abortions, malnutrition (the WHO estimates that a seventh of the global population, equivalent to 1 billion people, live in extreme poverty), as well as the number of armed conflicts and major disasters in the last 100 years are not a kind of "counterweight" to the also exponential growth of the global population. The two horrific World Wars in the last century caused the death of 100 million people alone, not including the victims of other "minor" military conflicts and tragedies such as the Holocaust in Germany, with 6 million victims, the twin towers in the USA, the Asian tsunami in the South of the Indian Ocean in December 2004, the frequent hurricanes and cyclones like Katrina at the end of August 2005, which caused losses of 45 billion US dollars, the Syrian conflict with more than one hundred thousand deaths and 4 million refugees, the death of some 60,000 people in the FARC & ELN guerrilla war in Colombia. The 150,000 deaths from violence in Venezuela in the last decade, in Cuba over 55 years with thousands of people being shot, dying in prison or dying when trying unsuccessfully to flee to exile, the no less devastating recent disaster in the Philippines and the birth restrictions in China. We might ask if the birth rate is growing at the same rate or in greater proportion to that of the mortality rate.

68th Paradox: Curative medicine vs. Preventative medicine

I would have to add that alcohol, drugs, tobacco, HIV, "junk" food, as well as starvation and malnutrition, a product of famine in Sudan and neighbouring regions, such as the poorest towns in India, China and Latin America, are all preventable causes of premature deaths in the world.

71st Paradox: Natural pharmaceutical products vs. Synthetic pharmaceuticals

The attitude demonstrated by third world governments in wasting the innumerable possibilities for conservation and health and life protection offered by international institutions (such as those mentioned in previous paradoxes) is completely irresponsible; this could be attributed to a type of inferiority complex, to ignorance or indifference to materials that are of such importance and of such high geo-human interest.

74th Paradox: Rural (and tropical) medicine vs. District community medicine

The solution to the problem continues to be high-quality and appropriate medical assistance in hospitals and health centres that are adequately supplied with sufficient and appropriate human resources, medical supplies and equipment, supplemented by a reliable and permanent educational prevention campaign, especially in rural areas.

76th Paradox: Diseases of deficiency vs. Diseases of affluence

I advise checking the Body Mass Index (ratio of weight in kg / height^2 in metres) to facilitate understanding. In the paradox where the volume of the USA population is mentioned, the figure should be updated; according to the latest census, the population is 330 million inhabitants.

84th Paradox: Chemical control of the risk factors of myocardial infarction and cerebrovascular accident vs. Treatment of already established diseases

If the patient afflicted by coronary or cardiovascular disease is successfully treated with specific pharmaceuticals that are administered separately, presumably the test "polypill", with its six ingredients, will achieve the same functions without significant reactions or rejections

320

in the long term. The issue lies in the dosage and frequency of ingestion, in view of the fact that the dosage and frequency of consumption of separately administered pharmaceuticals often varies according to the doctor's judgement. Medications like Losartan, Clopidogrel, Nimodipine and Simvastatin, amongst others, are dispensed in different dosages.

89th Paradox: Family medicine vs. Community medicine

The shaky, negative even, experience of the Barrio Adentro Mission demonstrates its clear weaknesses and failings, outweighing the socio-political benefits. Hence the need for a comprehensive reorganisation.

91st Paradox: The patient's decision vs. The treating doctors' decision

The responsibility is the treating doctor's, as long as the patient "approves" and complies with their prescriptions and instructions, and as long as the information they provide about their clinical history is complete, honest and true, with no hidden aspects that could have a negative impact on the diagnosis. As a general rule I write down my personal clinical history in advance of my annual and incidental check-ups, without omitting any details, and including previous conditions and any pharmaceuticals I am taking, in order to make my physician's job easier and keep them up-to-date in the case of an emergency. Generally, the medical questionnaire that the patient receives in their first consultation will be incomplete.

93rd Paradox: Medical novels vs. Medical autobiographies

In addition to what you have already established, I believe it is appropriate to dwell on the type and the frequency of TV and radio interviews with specialised doctors, which often turn into virtual "conferences" on their area of expertise. While this contributes to the imparting of medical knowledge and culture to the general public, it also runs the risk of misunderstandings, confusions, incorrect interpretations and the very common undesirable practice of self-medication and "recommendation" to other people afflicted with similar ills. In the majority of cases, these TV interviews conclude with the provision of the interviewee's details, address, telephone number and email address, at which point the interview simply turns into a long-duration advertisement.

Conclusion

I trust that these comments contribute in one way or another to the success of your "little book", which I do not hesitate to qualify as an excellent and useful essay-compilation of your extensive and diverse academic experience in the key fields of medical science; a contribution of singular importance for current and future generations.

Extracts from the speech about the author and the book given by
José Llort Brull on the occasion of the inauguration of
Dr Francisco Kerdel-Vegas into the Royal Academy
of Doctors in Spain
30 September 2014

ABOUT THE AUTHOR

Dr Francisco Kerdel-Vegas, born in Caracas, Venezuela on 3 January 1928, the son of Don Osvaldo Federico Kerdel and Doña Sofía Vegas, comes from a distinguished family of doctors. His maternal grandfather Dr Luis Vegas Sanabria was a doctor, two of his maternal uncles, Dr Martín Vegas, dermatologist and leprologist, and Dr Rafael Vegas, psychiatrist, and his eldest son Dr Francisco A. Kerdel is currently Professor of Dermatology at the University of Miami.

His primary and secondary education occurred in his birth city, first at the Instituto San Pablo and secondly at Liceo Andrés Bello. He began his professional training studying medicine at the Central University of Venezuela (1945–51), where he obtained the degree of Medical Surgeon. He interned at the Carlos J. Bello Red Cross Hospital in Venezuela and then travelled to the United States in order to specialise in Dermatology at the University of Harvard (Massachusetts General Hospital in Boston, 1951–52) and in New York University (Skin & Cancer Hospital of New York, 1952–54). In 1954 he was awarded the academic degree of Master of Science at New York University.

On returning to his country and desirous to follow in the footsteps of his maternal uncle Dr Martín Vegas, the father of Venezuelan Dermatology, he joined the Chair of Dermatology of the Faculty of Medicine at the Central University of Venezuela and the Dermatology Unit at the Hospital Vargas in Caracas as an Instructor, ascending through the years to the positions of Assistant Professor, Associate Professor and Professor. Within a very few years he obtained the degree of Doctor of Medical Sciences at the Central University of Venezuela.

He worked tirelessly alongside the illustrious dermatologist Professor Dr Jacinto Convit on projects that would lead to the establishment of the Institute of Dermatology, (today the Institute of Biomedicine, attached to the Hospital Vargas of Caracas), international recognition and the award of the first foreign donations for research into skin illnesses prevalent in the tropics. Ever since that time, the Hospital Vargas Dermatology Unit has been recognised by the American Board of Dermatology as one of the principal places in the world for the training of dermatologists. The Convit-Kerdel connection resulted in the discovery of two new skin diseases, *disseminated leishmaniasis* and *erythema dyschromicum perstans*. Alongside Professor Lewis Aronow of the University of Stanford, Dr Kerdel-Vegas also discovered the active ingredient (*seleno-cystathionine*) that produces hair loss caused by the ingestion of "Coco de Mono" seeds (*Lecythis ollaria*).

Dr Kerdel-Vegas moved to Great Britain during his sabbatical year in 1967, where he joined the University of Cambridge working on research at the Institute of Animal Physiology, Agricultural Research Council in Babraham near Cambridge, and with Dr Arthur Rook at Addenbrooke's Hospital. He was made a member of Trinity College, whilst simultaneously undertaking the role of Science attaché *ad honorem* to the Embassy of Venezuela in Great Britain.

During his time in Cambridge Dr Kerdel-Vegas established the *Cátedra Simón Bolívar de Estudios Latinoamericanos* (Simón Bolivar

Chair of Latin American Studies), financially supported by Shell of Venezuela, which has been running ever since.

On his return to Venezuela Dr Kerdel-Vegas founded the Andrés Bello Fellowship of studies on Venezuela at St Antony's College at the University of Oxford, with the support of the Venezuelan Central Bank. He also promoted the creation of eleven scholarships in perpetuity for Venezuelan students in different Colleges of the Universities of Cambridge and Oxford, which were established by the Academy of Physical Sciences, Mathematics and Natural Sciences (4 scholarships), the National Academy of Medicine (2), the Raúl Leoni Foundation (2), the Metropolitan University (1), the Boulton Foundation (1) and the Anala and Armando Planchart Foundation (1).

In 1967 he was elected a fellow of the Venezuelan National Academy of Medicine, and the following year he was invited to participate in a scientific expedition organised by the Armed Forces Institute of Pathology to Zaire (currently the Democratic Republic of Congo) to study in situ endemic diseases like Buruli ulcer and Onchocerciasis. In 1971, he was elected a fellow of the Venezuelan Academy of Physical Sciences, Mathematics and Natural Sciences.

He was also appointed Visiting Professor of Dermatology at the University of Columbia (New York) and of Jefferson Medical College (Philadelphia); he regularly visited both institutions and participated in their academic programmes for many years. He has been a frequent guest at the annual meetings of the American Academy of Dermatology where he has participated in and directed the Symposiums on Tropical Medicine. Other international affiliations include visiting Professor at the University of London (Institute of Dermatology at St Thomas' Hospital), fellow of the Philadelphia College of Physicians (Philadelphia) and the Royal Society of Medicine in London. He has been the Director of the *Acta Médica Venezolana*, the official body of Medical

Schools of the Federal District, and of the *Gaceta Médica de Caracas* (Caracas Medical Gazette), the oldest and most prestigious scientific journal in Venezuela and official publication of the National Academy of Medicine.

He actively participated in the creation of the Simón Bolívar University of Caracas, and once it was formally established he was appointed its first Academic Vice Chancellor. He also established and presided for many years over the National Committee of the United World Colleges in Venezuela, which selects Venezuelan students to be awarded a two-year scholarship in Colleges located in Wales, Canada, United States, Swaziland, Singapore, Italy, Hong Kong, Norway and India.

Dr Kerdel-Vegas aided HRH The Prince of Wales (then President of the United World Colleges) in the initiative to create the Simón Bolívar Agricultural College in Barinas; he was affiliated to that institution and worked as a member of its International Board for many years.

As a result of his great interest in conservation and nature he became involved in the creation of the *Fundación para la Defensa de la Naturaleza* or *FUDENA* (Foundation for the Defence of Nature), which is affiliated to the WWF in Switzerland. He was elected its first president and subsequently served for five years on the WWF International Board of Directors. In 1974 he was appointed CEO of the *Federación Panamericana de Facultades de Medicina* or *FEPAFEM* (Pan-American Federation of Faculties of Medicine) and it was his responsibility to relocate their Bogota offices to Caracas, acquiring the building that now houses their permanent headquarters.

In recognition of his pro-conservation activities and at the suggestion of Kathleen de Phelps, the ornithological society that she directed named a new species of hummingbird "Kerdel", this particular species of hummingbird, which was discovered in the Sierra de Turumiquire (between the states of Sucre and Monagas in Venezuela), was given the name *Thalsinus Kerdeli*. Years later that same hummingbird was chosen for the crest of the coat of arms awarded to him by the College of Arms in England.

Alongside Dr Federico Rivero Palacio, Dr Kerdel-Vegas approached the French and Venezuelan education authorities and took the necessary steps to establish in his own country an alternative system of superior education in order to sustain Venezuelan competitiveness in diverse sectors of the economy. The *Institutos Universitarios de Tecnología* (University Institutes of Technology) have worked very successfully for the last few decades.

He has been a member of the Jury of the prestigious Rolex Awards for entrepreneurial young people. He promoted the establishment of the International Foundation for Dermatology, formally created by the International League of Dermatological Societies in 1987, and has been part of its governing body for fifteen consecutive years since that time.

He actively participated in the recruitment process for the first dermatology training centres in two tropical countries most in need of these services, in the rural environments of Tanzania (Moshi) and Guatemala (Chimaltenango). This has resulted in the highly successful training of paramedics working in remote areas devoid of medical services.

Heeding the call to serve his country whenever the circumstances demanded it, in 1987 he accepted the nomination to serve as Ambassador to the United Kingdom of Great Britain and Northern Ireland, a position that he held until 1992. This new career separated him temporarily from the daily practice of dermatology, with which he tried to maintain academic contact. In 1994 he accepted the post of Ambassador and Permanent Delegate of Venezuela to UNESCO, and subsequently and simultaneously that of Ambassador to France, a position that he held until 1999.

There he continued his guiding work with young people, and with the support of UNESCO established the *Programa de Talento Venezolano en el exterior* or *TALVEN* (Venezuelan Talent Abroad Programme), which holds a database of more than a thousand experts and has arranged for more than 170 of them to visit Venezuela, thereby reconnecting with their country. The TALVEN programme was adopted in its day by the seven National Academies (Language, History, Medicine, Political & Social Sciences, Physical, Mathematical & Natural Sciences, Economic Sciences, and Engineering & Environment).

Dr Kerdel-Vegas has been the President of the Venezuelan Dermatology Society, and has won the prestigious Martín Vegas Prize twice, awarded by the Venezuelan Dermatology Society for the best work in that specialism. He is a Lifelong Member of the American Academy of Dermatology in the United States, and Honorary Member of the Dermatological Societies of Argentina, Germany, Austria, Brazil, Colombia, Costa Rica, Cuba, Ecuador, Spain, France, Mexico, Panama, Peru, Portugal, Puerto Rico, United Kingdom of Great Britain and Northern Ireland, the Dominican Republic and Uruguay. He is an Honorary Member of the National Academies of Medicine of Brazil, Colombia, Chile and Paraguay, Doctor of Sciences (Honorary) of Cranfield University (Great Britain) and of the San Francisco College of Podiatry.

He has won a number of important awards of which the following stand out:

> (In Venezuela) Order of the Liberator, Order of Francisco de Miranda, Order of Andrés Bello, Order of Cecilio Acosta, Order of Diego de Losada, Sun of Carabobo Order, Order of Merit at Work, Order of Henri Pittier, The Venezuelan Medical Federation Francisco Herrera Luque Medal

(Abroad) Commander of the British Empire (CBE), Knight of the National Order of the Legion of Honour and Grand Officer of The National Order of Merit (France)

He has written numerous books on dermatology, is the co-author of an important treatise on dermatology, and in collaboration with the eminent dermatologist Dr George Clinton Andrews is the author of the work *Enfermedades de la Piel* (Skin Diseases).

He recently worked on a programme intended to lead to an information revolution in the poorest sectors of the population, via the use of computers and access to the Internet.

MEDICAL PARADOXES

Dr Kerdel-Vegas' Medical Paradoxes is of such great practical importance that it should form part of the medical curriculum, especially when students begin to make contact with their first patients and the illnesses that afflict them. It is the embodiment of moderation and good advice, an antidote to the omnipotence that so often embraces modern medicine, which is so dazzled by technology; it will help to redress the balance between them. It reflects not only that Dr Kerdel-Vegas is first and foremost a great doctor, but much more. He possesses those spiritual and other qualities that encapsulate everything a doctor should be, not just a craftsman of medicine but a person of great literary and scientific culture, of life wisdom, a literate man and a humanist.

Medical Paradoxes acknowledges that the daily practice of medicine presents numerous contradictions that are difficult to interpret and even more complex to resolve. The various paradoxes chosen at random and in no way a complete inventory encompass a variety of aspects: philosophical, ethical, moral, ontological, deontological, semiological, semantic, economic, administrative, procedural, cultural amongst others, but what they have in common is an interest of a practical nature for the doctor in the practice of his or her profession.

I conclude by quoting the brief but suitable and illustrative words written about *Medical Paradoxes* by the eminent ophthalmologist Dr Arturo Ramos Caldera:

> "Reading the book was thrilling, entertaining and interesting, which is why I believe its publication will fill an important gap in the overall training of all students of medicine. Even when an in-depth analysis of each and every one of its topics is not attempted (which would be impossible to achieve), the simple act of listing them and of citing a bibliography for each one offers an overall view for the reader and a first guide to dig deeper into those that most interest them."

INDEX

346

347